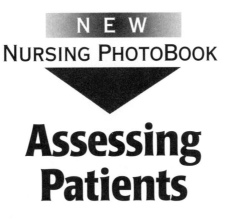

NEW
NURSING PHOTOBOOK

Assessing Patients

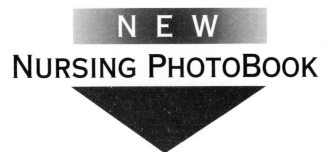

NEW
NURSING PHOTOBOOK

Assessing Patients

Springhouse Corporation
Springhouse, Pennsylvania

STAFF

Senior Publisher
Matthew Cahill

Clinical Manager
Cindy Tryniszewski, RN, MSN

Art Director
John Hubbard

Senior Editor
June Norris

Clinical Editors
Judith Schilling McCann, RN, BSN (clinical project editor), Beverly Tscheschlog, RN

Editor
Elizabeth Weinstein

Copy Editors
Cynthia C. Breuninger (manager), Lynette High, Doris Weinstock

Designers
Stephanie Peters (senior associate art director), Lorraine Carbo, Darcy Feralio

Photographer
John Gallagher

Typographers
Diane Paluba (manager), Elizabeth Bergman, Joyce Rossi Biletz, Phyllis Marron, Valerie Rosenberger

Manufacturing
Deborah Meiris (director), Pat Dorshaw (manager), T.A. Landis

Production Coordinator
Margaret A. Rastiello

Editorial Assistants
Beverly Lane, Mary Madden

Indexer
Barbara Hodgson

The clinical procedures described and recommended in this publication are based on research and consultation with nursing, medical, and legal authorities. To the best of our knowledge, these procedures reflect currently accepted practice; nevertheless, they can't be considered absolute and universal recommendations. For individual application, all recommendations must be considered in light of the patient's clinical condition and, before administration of new or infrequently used drugs, in light of the latest package insert information. The authors and the publisher disclaim responsibility for any adverse effects resulting directly or indirectly from the suggested procedures, from any undetected errors, or from the reader's misunderstanding of the text.

Printed in the United States of America

A member of the Reed Elsevier plc group

PHOBK1-010795

Library of Congress Cataloging-in-Publication Data
Assessing patients.
p. cm. — (New nursing photobooks)
Includes index.
1. Nursing assessment. 2. Physical diagnosis.
I. Springhouse Corporation. II. Series
[DNLM: 1. Nursing Assessment—methods.
WY 100.4 A846 1996]
RT48.A83 1996
616.70'5—dc20
DNLM/DLC 95-6497
ISBN 0-87434-808-0 CIP

CONTENTS

FOREWORD

Excellent assessment skills have always been a cornerstone of good nursing practice. And they remain so today, even as patients are admitted to the hospital only when strict criteria are met and are discharged to outpatient settings much earlier than in the past. Knowing which questions to ask, really hearing what a patient tells you about his chief complaint, and conducting a thorough but efficient physical examination goes a long way toward achieving the best possible outcome for every patient.

In *Assessing Patients,* you'll find over 400 step-by-step photographs that actually *show* you every important technique in a head-to-toe nursing assessment. From taking a health history to performing a physical examination, each assessment technique is presented in photographs or in meticulous, detailed illustrations, or both.

Extremely versatile, *Assessing Patients* is divided into two major sections: "Understanding Assessment" and "Assessing the Body." Read it straight through—from "Learning about Assessment" to "Examining Peripheral Circulation"—or pick it up for a quick consultation before making a cardiac or sensorimotor assessment, for example.

You'll find the text highly readable. Concise directions eliminate the need to wade through wordy descriptions of assessment steps. To introduce you to each assessment, you'll first find a discussion with photos of anatomy and physiology. Following this, an *Assessment checklist* reminds you which history question to ask. Next follows detailed assessment steps, with each step accompanied by close-up, detailed photographs. The photographs are easy to follow and clinically accurate; they're the next best thing to having an expert nurse at your elbow.

A number of extra features enhance this book's usefulness and make it an essential tool for the busiest nurse. Look for graphic devices, or logos, which highlight valuable information. For instance, *Clinical tips* point out ways to perform a step more efficiently or to use an alternative method. *Insights and interpretations* provides an in-depth view of physical examination findings; for example, when examining the abdomen, this feature tells you what abdominal and bowel sounds signify, where they're located, and what causes them.

No matter what setting you work in and whether you see 5 or 50 patients a day, I know you'll find *Assessing Patients* an indispensable guide in your nursing practice.

Cathy Sellergren, RN, MSN, CCRN
Pulmonary Case Manager
Hinsdale Hospital, Ill

Understanding Assessment

LEARNING ABOUT ASSESSMENT

Whether you're briefly checking your patient's over-all appearance or fully exploring his chief complaint, you're performing a part of an assessment. Knowing how to carry out an accurate assessment—from taking a health history through performing a physical examination—will help you uncover important problems and direct your care.

TAKING A HEALTH HISTORY

A thorough health history allows you to identify the patient's specific health problems. Take a holistic approach. Combine general information with the patient's chief complaint, review past health patterns and present illness, and evaluate the patient's response to his current condition. Of course, you'll need to establish an atmosphere of trust and rapport so that the patient can frankly and comfortably convey information. (See *Guidelines for an effective interview*.)

A complete health history covers biographical data, the patient's chief complaint, his medical history (including all medications—past and present, prescription and nonprescription), family history, psychosocial history (including data on activities of daily living), and a review of body systems. If your patient is young, elderly, or unable to communicate, you may need to obtain the history from a parent or other relative, a friend, or a caregiver.

Biographical data

Begin the history by recording the patient's name, address, age, birth date, and birthplace. Also record his race, nationality, religion, present and previous occupations, and marital status. Ask about family members or other persons with whom he lives, and obtain the name, address, and phone number of a responsible person to contact in an emergency. Also ask the patient to identify his doctor or other usual health care provider. If the patient can't give accurate information, obtain data from a relative or friend. Document who provided the information.

Chief complaint

Ask the patient why he's seeking health care, and record his exact words in quotation marks. Find out how and when his symptoms developed and how they affect his life-style. Thoroughly investigate each symptom to ensure that you collect all pertinent data.

To remember what information you need, use the PQRST mnemonic device. Begin with *P* and progress to *T.*

P for provocative or palliative
• Ask what provokes or relieves the symptom.
• Does an activity trigger the symptom?
• Do recognizable factors, such as stress, anger, or physical position, cause the symptom to occur?
• What makes the symptom worsen or subside?

Q for quality and quantity
• Ask what the symptom feels, looks, or sounds like. Have the patient describe it fully.
• How much of the symptom is the patient experiencing currently? Is this more or less than usual?
• To what degree does the symptom affect normal activities?

R for region and radiation
• Ask where in the body the symptom occurs.
• Does it radiate to other regions? If so, which areas?

S for severity
• Ask about the symptom's severity. Have the patient rate severity on a scale of 1 to 10, with 10 being the most severe.
• Does the symptom seem to be diminishing, intensifying, or unchanging?

T for timing
• Ask the patient when the symptom began.
• Was the onset sudden or gradual?
• How often does the patient experience the symptom?
• How long does the symptom last?

Medical history
Ask the patient about previous illnesses, injuries, and immunizations. Note the dates of significant treatments and surgeries and when and why he last sought medical treatment.

Teresa Palmer, RN, CANP, MSN, contributed to this section. She is a clinical assistant professor at the University of Medicine and Dentistry, New Brunswick, N.J., and a nurse practitioner in adult cardiac surgery at the Robert Wood Johnson University Hospital in New Brunswick. The publisher also thanks the following organizations for their help: *Critikon,* Tampa, Fla.; *Delcrest Medical,* Blue Bell, Pa.; *Doylestown (Pa.) Hospital; Hill Rom,* Batesville, Ind.; *IVAC Corp.,* San Diego, Calif.; *Pymah Corp.,* Somerville, N.J.; and *Village Pharmacy at Springhouse,* Springhouse, Pa.

Guidelines for an effective interview

Developing an effective interviewing technique will help you collect pertinent health history information efficiently. Use the following guidelines to enhance your interviewing skills.

Be prepared
• Review all available information before the interview. Read current clinical records and, if applicable, previous records ahead of time. This will help you focus the interview, prevent tiring the patient, and save you time.
• Remember to review with the patient what you've learned to be sure the information is correct. Keep in mind that the patient's current complaint may be unrelated to his history.

Create a pleasant interviewing atmosphere
• Be sure to select a quiet, well-lighted, and relaxed setting. Keep in mind that extraneous noise and activity can interfere with concentration, as can excessive or insufficient light. You should strive for a relaxed atmosphere, which eases the patient's anxiety, promotes comfort, and conveys your willingness to listen.
• Ensure privacy. Some patients won't share personal information if they suspect that others can overhear. You may, however, let friends or family members remain if the patient requests it or if he needs their help.
• Make sure the patient feels as comfortable as possible. If the patient is too tired, short of breath, or frightened, you should provide care and reschedule the history taking.
• Take your time. If you appear rushed, you may distract the patient. Assure the patient that he has your undivided attention; then listen attentively. If you have little time, you should focus on specific interest areas and return later instead of hurrying through the entire interview.

Establish a good rapport
• Sit and chat for a few minutes with the patient before the interview. Standing may suggest that you're in a hurry and lead the patient to rush, omitting important information.
• Be sure to explain the interview's purpose. Emphasize how the patient benefits when the health care team has the information needed to diagnose and treat a disorder.
• Show your concern for the patient's story. Maintain eye contact, and occasionally repeat what he tells

you. If you seem preoccupied or disinterested, he may choose not to confide in you.
• Encourage the patient to help you develop a plan of care that will serve his perceived needs and that is realistic.

Set the tone and focus
• Encourage the patient to talk about his chief complaint. This helps you focus on his most troublesome signs and symptoms and provides an opportunity to assess the patient's emotional state and level of understanding.
• Be sure to keep the interview informal but professional. Allow the patient time to answer questions fully and add his own perceptions. When necessary, however, you should redirect the conversation to the main subject.
• Speak clearly and simply. Avoid using medical terms because the patient may not tell you that he doesn't understand them.
• Be sure that the patient understands you. If you think he doesn't, you should have him restate what you've talked about.
• Pay close attention to the patient's words and actions, interpreting not only what he says but also what he doesn't say.

Choose your words carefully
• Ask open-ended questions to encourage the patient to provide complete and pertinent information. Questions that require only a yes-or-no answer may discourage him from elaborating.
• Listen carefully to the patient's answers. Use his words in your subsequent questions to encourage his elaboration on his signs, symptoms, and other problems.

Take notes
• Avoid documenting all the information during the interview, but make sure you jot down important information, such as dates, times, and key words or phrases. Use these to help you recall the complete history for the medical record.

Surveying activities of daily living

A record of the patient's daily activities—diet and elimination patterns, exercise and sleep habits, work and leisure activities, and other factors, such as tobacco and alcohol use—can provide a comprehensive view of his life-style. To learn as much as possible, ask these questions.

Diet and elimination
- [ ] How would you describe your appetite?
- [ ] What do you normally eat in a day?
- [ ] What do you like and dislike to eat? Is your diet restricted in any way?
- [ ] How much fluid do you drink during an average day?
- [ ] Are you allergic to any foods?
- [ ] When do you usually go to the bathroom? Has this schedule changed recently?
- [ ] Do you take any foods, fluids, or drugs to help you maintain your normal elimination (bowel and bladder) patterns?

Exercise and sleep
- [ ] Do you have a special exercise program? What kind? How long have you been following it? How do you feel after exercising?
- [ ] How many hours do you sleep each day? When? Do you feel rested afterward?
- [ ] What do you do to help you fall asleep?
- [ ] What do you do when you can't sleep?
- [ ] Do you wake up during the night?
- [ ] Do you have sleepy spells during the day? When?
- [ ] Do you take naps routinely?

Work and leisure
- [ ] What do you do when you're at work (or school or home)?
- [ ] What kind of unpaid work do you do for enjoyment?
- [ ] How much leisure time do you have?
- [ ] How do you spend your leisure time?
- [ ] In what ways do you and your family share leisure time?
- [ ] How do your weekends differ from your weekdays?

Tobacco, alcohol, and other drugs
- [ ] Do you use tobacco? What kind do you use? How much do you use each day? Each week? How long have you used it? Have you ever tried to stop using it?
- [ ] Do you drink alcohol? If so, how much do you drink each day? Each week? What time of the day do you usually drink?
- [ ] What kind of alcohol (beer, wine, hard liquor) do you drink?
- [ ] Do you usually drink alone or with others?
- [ ] Do you drink more when you feel stressed?
- [ ] In what ways, if any, does drinking affect your job or school performance?
- [ ] Do you or your family ever worry about your drinking?
- [ ] Do you feel dependent on alcohol, coffee, tea, or soft drinks? How much of these beverages do you drink in an average day?
- [ ] Can you name the prescription drugs you take? Nonprescription drugs?
- [ ] Do you use any illicit drugs, such as marijuana or cocaine? If you do, how often do you use them?

Find out if the patient has allergies—particularly to medications, such as antibiotics. Ask about prescription and nonprescription medications he uses.

Family history

Ask the patient about the health of his family. Find out, for example, if any family members had or have cancer or diabetes mellitus. Also ask if any family members have unusual limitations (such as paralysis from a cerebrovascular accident).

Psychosocial history

Have the patient describe his usual activities of daily living and whether these activities have changed in response to his chief complaint. Discuss diet and elimination patterns, exercise and sleep patterns, recreation, and use of alcohol, tobacco, and other drugs. (See *Surveying activities of daily living.*)

Assess how the patient feels about himself and how he views his position in the community and his relationships with others. Ask about his occupation, education, financial status, and responsibilities.

Evaluate the patient's coping strategies. Ask how he has dealt with past medical, emotional, or social crises. Investigate recent changes in his life-style, personality, or behavior.

Body systems review

After you've collected these data, review common symptoms in each body system. (For guidelines see *Reviewing body structures and systems.*)

ASSESSMENT CHECKLIST

Reviewing body structures and systems

When you're collecting information about the patient's condition, you'll need to systematically assess body structures and systems. In this checklist, you'll find key questions to ask about each structure and system.

Overall health

☐ Ask the patient if he has noticed changes in his weight. Do his clothes, rings, or shoes fit more tightly than usual?

☐ Does he have nonspecific symptoms, such as weakness, fatigue, or fever?

☐ Can he keep up with normal daily activities?

Skin

☐ Ask the patient to describe any changes in skin pigmentation, temperature, moisture, or hair distribution.

☐ Find out if the patient has rashes, lesions, itching, or scaling. Is his skin excessively dry or oily?

☐ Has the patient noticed easy bruising or bleeding, changes in warts or moles, lumps, or changes in hair or nails?

Head

☐ Has the patient experienced a head injury?

☐ Does the patient have alopecia or any lumps on his head?

☐ Does the patient get headaches? If so, how often do they occur? Has the patient identified a precipitating cause? How long do the headaches last? What relieves the headaches? What makes them worse?

Neck

☐ Investigate neck problems—pain, swelling, stiffness, lumps, swollen glands, goiter, or limited movement.

☐ If the patient has a neck problem, ask when it occurred. Was it precipitated by a particular incident? Does anything ease or exacerbate it?

☐ If the patient has neck pain, does it radiate to or from another part of the body? Have the patient describe the pain. Is it constant or intermittent?

Nose

☐ Explore the patient's nasal problems, including sinusitis, discharge, colds, coryza (more than four times a year), rhinitis, trauma, or frequent sneezing.

☐ Does he have an obstruction, breathing problems, or an inability to smell? Has he had nosebleeds?

☐ Has the patient ever had any surgery on his nose or sinuses? If so, explore when and why the surgery was done and what type of procedure was done.

Mouth and throat

☐ Investigate whether the patient has sores in the mouth or on the tongue. Does he have toothaches, bleeding gums, loss of taste, voice changes, dry mouth, or frequent sore throats?

☐ If the patient has frequent sore throats, when do they occur? Are they associated with fever or difficulty swallowing? How have the sore throats been treated medically?

☐ Has the patient ever had a problem swallowing? If so, does he have trouble swallowing solids or liquids? Is the problem constant or intermittent? What precipitates the swallowing difficulty? What makes it go away?

☐ Does he have dental caries or tooth loss? Ask if he wears dentures.

Eyes

☐ Ask the patient about visual problems, such as myopia, hyperopia, blurred vision, or double vision. Does he wear corrective lenses?

☐ Does he have a history of glaucoma, cataracts, or other eye disorders?

☐ Does he experience excessive tearing, dry eyes, itching, burning, pain, inflammation, swelling, color blindness, or photophobia?

☐ When was his last eye examination?

Ears

☐ Does the patient have hearing problems, such as deafness, poor hearing, tinnitus, or vertigo? Does he wear a hearing aid?

☐ Find out if he has ear discharge, pain, or tenderness behind the ears.

☐ Inquire about frequent or recent ear infection or ear surgery.

Respiratory system

☐ Inquire about dyspnea, shortness of breath, pain, wheezing, paroxysmal nocturnal dyspnea, and orthopnea (number of pillows used).

☐ Review whether the patient experiences cough, sputum production, hemoptysis, or night sweats.

☐ Does he have emphysema, pleurisy, bronchitis, tuberculosis, pneumonia, asthma, or frequent respiratory infections?

☐ What are the dates and results of the patient's last chest X-ray and tuberculin skin test?

(continued)

Reviewing body structures and systems *(continued)*

Cardiovascular system
☐ Ask about cardiac problems, such as palpitations, tachycardia or other irregular rhythms, chest pain, dyspnea on exertion, paroxysmal nocturnal dyspnea, orthopnea, and cough.
☐ Explore vascular problems. Does the patient experience cyanosis, edema, ascites, intermittent claudication, cold extremities, or phlebitis?
☐ Ask the patient about postural hypotension, hypertension, rheumatic fever, varicose veins, and peripheral vascular disease.
☐ When (if ever) did the patient have his last electrocardiogram?

Breasts
☐ In women, inquire about changes in breast development or lactation patterns, mastitis history, nipple discharge, and a history of breast cancer. Does the patient perform breast self-examination?
☐ In men, ask about gynecomastia.
☐ In women and men, check for trauma, pain, lumps, and changes in breast contour.

GI system
☐ Explore signs and symptoms. For example, find out about appetite and weight changes, dysphagia, nausea, vomiting, heartburn, stomach or abdominal pain, frequent belching or flatulence, hematemesis, and jaundice.
☐ Does the patient use laxatives frequently? Ask about hemorrhoids, rectal bleeding, character of stools (color, odor, and consistency), and changes in bowel habits.
☐ Has he had hernias, gallbladder disease, or liver disease, such as hepatitis?

Renal and genitourinary systems
☐ Inquire about urine color, polyuria, oliguria, and nocturia (number of urinations per night). Does the patient experience incontinence, dysuria, frequency, urgency, or difficulty with urinary stream (such as reduced flow or dribbling)?
☐ Find out about pyuria, urine retention, or passage of calculi.

Reproductive system
☐ In men, ask about penile discharge or lesions and testicular pain or lumps. Does the patient perform testicular self-examination? Has he had a vasectomy?

☐ In females, ask about age at onset of menarche and the character of menstrual periods (frequency, regularity, and duration). When was the patient's last menstrual period? Does she have irregular or painful vaginal bleeding, dyspareunia, or frequent vaginal infections? Ask the patient about the character of pregnancies (number, durations, deliveries, and abortions, either spontaneous or induced), birth control methods, and age at menopause. What was the date of the patient's last gynecologic examination and Pap test?
☐ In men and women, ask about sexually transmitted diseases and other infections.

Musculoskeletal system
☐ Does the patient experience muscle pain, joint pain, swelling, tenderness, back problems, or difficulty with balance or gait? In addition, find out about injuries, weakness, paralysis, deformities, or limited motion.
☐ Does the patient have arthritis or gout?

Neurologic system
☐ Investigate the character of any headaches (frequency, intensity, location, and duration).
☐ Does the patient have seizures, vertigo, syncope, tremors, twitching, numbness and tingling, aphasia, weakness, paralysis, loss of sensation, or disequilibrium?

Hematopoietic system
☐ Does the patient have anemia or bleeding abnormalities? Does he experience excessive fatigue or easy bruising?
☐ Has he undergone transfusions? What were his reactions to them?

Endocrine and metabolic systems
☐ Explore signs and symptoms, such as polyuria, polydipsia, excessive sweating, and changes in hair distribution and amount.
☐ Ask about nervousness, diabetes, goiter, recent weight change, and heat or cold intolerance. Assess for neck swelling.

Mental health
☐ Inquire about mood changes, anxiety, depression, inability to concentrate or cope, stress, and memory loss.

STARTING THE PHYSICAL EXAMINATION

As the first step in the physical examination, the general survey provides important information about the patient's overall health status.

GENERAL SURVEY

This survey requires skilled, focused observations and a confident, professional approach.

First, observe the patient for signs of physical or emotional distress. Then proceed to note facial characteristics, body type, posture, movement, voice and speech, general appearance, and psychological state. Summarize your findings in a brief paragraph.

• *Physical or emotional distress.* Note whether the patient appears ill and needs immediate attention. Observe his mental status and general demeanor. Is he alert? Is he in pain? Is he dyspneic? Does he appear agitated or have difficulty listening to you?

• *Facial characteristics.* Check the patient's facial expression. Does it portray tension? Is his expression appropriate for the situation? Does he look older or younger than his stated age?

• *Body type.* Classify the patient as stocky, average, or slender. Is he cachetic or obese? Does he have a barrel chest? Do you see finger clubbing, edema, or joint contractures?

• *Posture.* Note whether the patient stands erect and whether his body is symmetrical. Remember that minor variations are normal.

• *Movement.* When the patient walks, observe his coordination and gait. If he's in bed, can he turn, sit up, and reposition himself? Does he lean forward to breathe?

• *Voice and speech.* Listen to the patient's vocal tone and clarity. Also note vocal strength. Is he hoarse? Can the patient articulate and communicate verbally? Note, too, the patient's vocabulary and word usage.

• *General appearance.* What's the general condition of the patient's clothes? Are they seasonally appropriate? Do you smell odors, such as alcohol, urine, or excessive cologne? Does the patient seem concerned about his appearance? Can he care for himself?

When making clinical judgments about the patient's appearance, be sure to consider the impact of the patient's culture, educational level, socioeconomic status, and recent life experiences.

• *Psychological state.* Assess the patient's level of consciousness, awareness, attentiveness, attention span, and orientation. Can he follow simple instructions? Does he appear relaxed and comfortable, or nervous and fidgety? Does he have any bizarre mannerisms? Note, too, whether the patient has any unusual features.

BASELINE DATA: HEIGHT, WEIGHT, AND VITAL SIGNS

Besides recording your general observations, you'll need to compile baseline measurements of the patient's height and weight. In addition, take his vital signs.

Measuring the patient's height

The height-weight ratio serves as a starting point for evaluating current health status. You'll measure the patient's height in inches (or centimeters) with a wall-mounted measuring stick or the measuring bar on a standard standing scale (as shown below at left).

▶ *Clinical tip:* If you use a movable standing scale, be sure to lock the wheels before the patient gets on the scale.

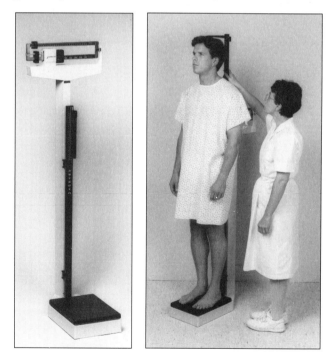

An older child or an adult who can stand without support should remove his shoes and stand erect on the scale. Then ask the patient to look straight ahead.

Raise the L-shaped measuring bar above the patient's head. Extend the horizontal arm, and lower it until it rests atop the patient's head (as shown above at right).

Desirable weight ranges for adults

Healthful weight ranges depend on an adult's height and age. Use the information below to assess your patient's height-weight ratio. The higher weights in each range typically apply to men, who have more muscle and bone; lower weights usually apply to women, who have less muscle and bone. Suggested weights for people age 35 and over are higher than those for younger adults. This reflects recent findings that older people can carry somewhat more weight without impairing their health.

HEIGHT	WEIGHT (LB)		HEIGHT	WEIGHT (LB)	
	Ages 19 to 34	Ages 35 and over		Ages 19 to 34	Ages 35 and over
5'0"	97 to 128	108 to 138	5'10"	132 to 174	146 to 188
5'1"	101 to 132	111 to 143	5'11"	136 to 179	151 to 194
5'2"	104 to 137	115 to 148	6'0"	140 to 184	155 to 199
5'3"	107 to 141	119 to 152	6'1"	144 to 189	159 to 205
5'4"	111 to 146	122 to 157	6'2"	148 to 195	164 to 210
5'5"	114 to 150	126 to 162	6'3"	152 to 200	168 to 216
5'6"	118 to 155	130 to 167	6'4"	156 to 205	173 to 222
5'7"	121 to 160	134 to 172	6'5"	160 to 211	177 to 228
5'8"	125 to 164	138 to 178	6'6"	164 to 216	182 to 234
5'9"	129 to 169	142 to 183			

Source: U.S. Department of Agriculture, U.S. Department of Health and Human Services. *Nutrition and Your Health: Dietary Guidelines for Americans*, 3rd ed. Washington, D.C., 1990.

Now read and record the patient's height shown by the measuring bar.

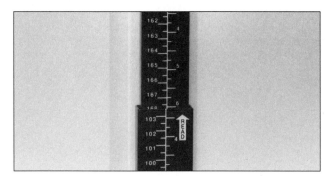

Weighing the patient

Along with height, the patient's weight is essential for assessing nutritional status; calculating dosages of medications, anesthetics, and contrast media; and determining the height-weight ratio. (See *Desirable weight ranges for adults*.)

By monitoring the patient's weight, you may also detect the onset of some disorders, such as heart failure or excessive diuresis. When you need precise measurements, use the same scale each time. Weigh the patient at the same time and in similar, lightweight clothing each day. When using a movable scale, be sure to lock the wheels before proceeding.

To weigh the patient on a standing scale, ask him to remove his shoes and step onto the scale. Tell him to center his feet on the platform. Locate the movable weights that ride across a two-part, horizontal balance bar atop the standard scale. The bars are joined in an arrow-shaped arrangement that balances in a frame. The arrow rises and falls with the position of the weights but levels off when the patient's weight and the scale weights are matched. The balance bar is notched. Grooves in the lower bar represent 50, 100, 150, and 200 lb; grooves in the upper bar measure quarters of a pound. Now slide the lower weight into the groove representing the largest increment below the patient's estimated weight. For example, if you think the patient weighs

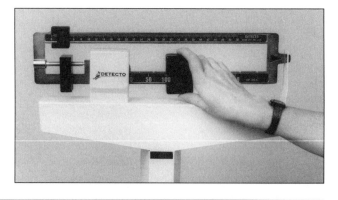

How age affects vital signs

Normal vital signs vary with the patient's age. The chart below shows appropriate ranges for patients of all ages.

AGE (YR)	TEMPERATURE	RESTING PULSE RATE (BEATS/MINUTE)		RESPIRATORY RATE (BREATHS/MINUTE)	MEAN BLOOD PRESSURE
		Average	Normal range		
Infant	97° to 100° F axillary (36.1° to 37.8° C)	125	70 to 190	30 to 80	78 systolic 42 diastolic 30/60 by flush technique
1	99.7° F (37.6° C) rectal	120	80 to 160	20 to 40	96 systolic 65 diastolic
2	98.9° F (37.2° C) rectal	120	80 to 160	20 to 40	100 systolic 63 diastolic
4	Same	100	80 to 120	20 to 30	97 systolic 64 diastolic
6	96.7° to 99.5° F (35.9° to 37.5° C)	100	75 to 115	20 to 25	98 systolic 65 diastolic
8	Same	90	70 to 110	20 to 25	106 systolic 70 diastolic
10	Same	90	70 to 110	17 to 22	110 systolic 72 diastolic
12	Same	Male: 85 Female: 90	65 to 105 70 to 110	17 to 22	116 systolic 74 diastolic
14	Same	Male: 80 Female: 85	60 to 100 60 to 100	15 to 20	120 systolic 76 diastolic
16	Same	Male: 75 Female: 80	55 to 95 60 to 100	15 to 20	123 systolic 76 diastolic
18	Same	Male: 70 Female: 75	50 to 90 55 to 95	15 to 20	126 systolic 79 diastolic
19 to 69	Same	Same as age 18	Same as age 18	15 to 20	120 systolic 80 diastolic
70 and over	96.7° F (36° C)	Same as age 18	Same as age 18	15 to 20	Diastolic pressure may increase.

145 lb, slide the rider into the groove for 100 lb. Slide the upper weight across the bar until the bar balances parallel to the floor. Add the numbers designated by the lower and upper weights. The sum is the patient's weight to the nearest quarter of a pound.

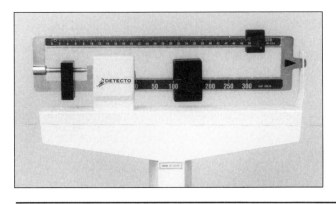

Record the patient's weight and help him off the scale. Then return the scale weights to their original positions, and return the scale to its proper place.

Assessing vital signs

Taking vital signs, a routine nursing function, provides important information about the patient's current health and serves as a baseline for subsequent measurements. During the initial examination, you'll record the patient's temperature, resting pulse rate, respiratory rate, and blood pressure. Then you'll take these vital signs again at regular intervals: every 4 to 6 hours for a hospitalized patient, every 1 to 2 hours for a patient in critical condition, and as often as every 15 minutes for a patient who has just undergone surgery or another invasive procedure.

Types of thermometers

You can take an oral, rectal, or axillary temperature with such instruments as a mercury glass thermometer, a chemical dot device, or various electronic digital thermometers. You may even have access to a tympanic thermometer.

You'll use the oral route most for adults who are awake, alert, oriented, and cooperative. For infants, young children, and confused or unconscious patients, you may need to take the temperature rectally.

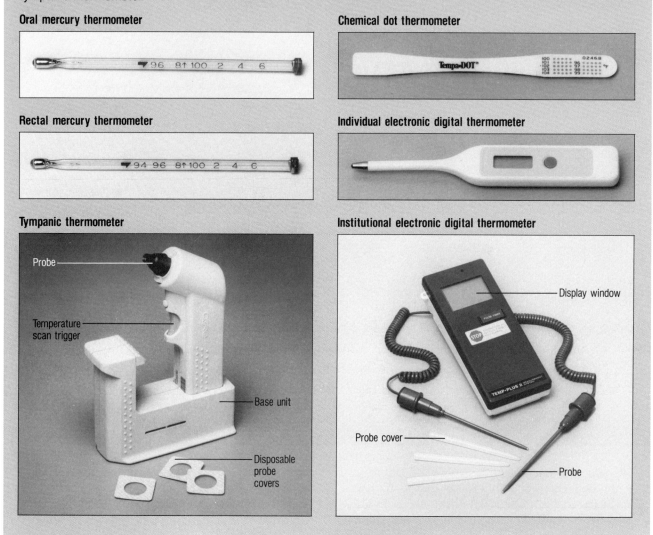

Oral mercury thermometer

Rectal mercury thermometer

Tympanic thermometer

Probe

Temperature scan trigger

Base unit

Disposable probe covers

Chemical dot thermometer

Individual electronic digital thermometer

Institutional electronic digital thermometer

Display window

Probe cover

Probe

Although your initial measurements can alert you to problems that need immediate attention, serial readings provide even more valuable information. Two or more abnormal vital signs may signal a beginning or worsening disorder, so always analyze a series of vital signs, not just the latest readings.

Physical or emotional stress can alter vital signs also, so help the patient to relax before you begin. If you obtain an abnormal value, take the vital sign again. For an abnormal blood pressure, have the patient lie down for a while, then retake the measure-

ment. Remember that normal readings vary with the patient's age. (See *How age affects vital signs.*)

Taking the patient's temperature

Temperature is the difference between the amount of body heat produced and the amount of body heat lost. Recorded in degrees Fahrenheit (F) or degrees Celsius (C), normal body temperature ranges from 96.7° to 99.5° F (35.9° to 37.5° C), depending on how it's measured (see *Types of thermometers*). Normal temperature also varies with age, sex, physi-

Taking tympanic membrane temperature

The tympanic thermometer computes body temperature electronically with a pluglike probe that you insert gently in the ear. The probe responds quickly to subtle thermal changes and registers a value accurately. Here's how to use it:
• Lift the probe from the base unit.
• Cap the probe with the disposable cover.
• Insert the probe deep enough in the ear canal to seal the opening.

▶ **Clinical tip:** When inserting the probe, avoid tugging on the ear to straighten the ear canal. Recent studies indicate that tugging may lower temperature readings slightly.
• Press the trigger to start the temperature scan.
• Listen for the beep that signals a completed temperature reading (in a few seconds).
• Record the displayed temperature.
• Remove and discard the probe cover.
• Return the probe to the base unit.

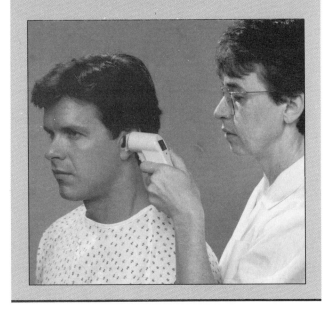

cal activity, and environment. What's more, temperature changes may occur with metabolic diseases (such as hyperthyroidism), severe infection, myocardial infarction, and surgery.

Depending on your workplace, you may use traditional devices, such as a glass thermometer, or more sophisticated ones, such as a tympanic membrane thermometer. (For more information, see *Taking tympanic membrane temperature*.) Typically, though, you'll use an electronic digital thermometer.

Although this thermometer is expensive initially, it's fast, easy to use, and accurate. Equipped with two probes (a blue-topped one for oral temperature and a red-topped one for rectal temperature), the electronic digital thermometer is portable and easily stored. Before using an electronic digital oral thermometer, be sure it's fully charged and calibrated.

To begin, remove the thermometer from its rechargeable stand. Be sure that the top of the temperature probe is blue. Then insert the thermometer probe into a disposable plastic cover. Position the tip of the covered probe under the patient's tongue and as far back as possible, on either side of the frenulum linguae. Have the patient close his lips around the thermometer, but caution him not to bite it.

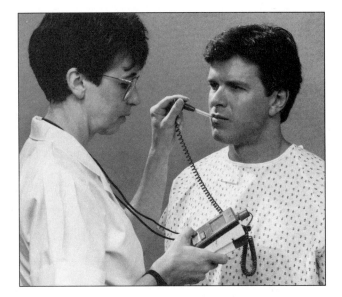

When the probe finishes measuring the patient's temperature—usually in 10 to 30 seconds—you'll hear a beep and see the temperature value displayed digitally on a screen. When this happens, remove the thermometer, discard the disposable probe cover, and return the device to the stand.

Taking the patient's pulse

Pulse rate reflects the rhythmic expansion of the arteries as the heart ejects blood with each beat. To assess the patient's pulse, you'll note the rhythm, rate, and amplitude of the beat as you palpate or auscultate over a pulse point. (See *Locating pulse sites*, page 12.)

Palpate the most accessible site—the radial pulse—with the pads of your index and middle fingers (not your thumb, which has its own pulse). In a cardiovascular crisis, you may palpate pulses over the femoral and carotid arteries. Because these arteries are larger and closer to the heart, they more

Locating pulse sites

You can assess your patient's pulse rate at several sites, which are shown below. The site you select depends on various factors, such as the patient's condition.

Brachial pulse

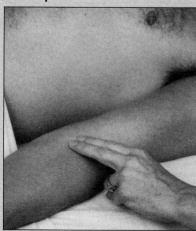

Radial pulse

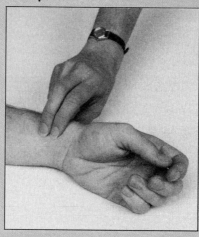

Carotid pulse

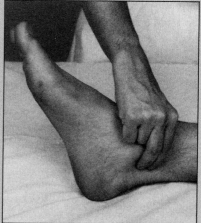

Femoral pulse

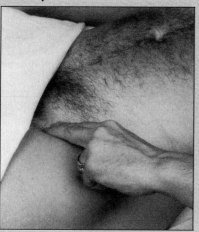

Pedal pulse

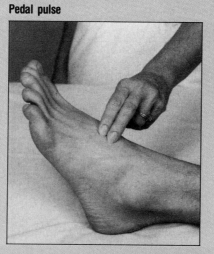

Posterior tibial pulse

Popliteal pulse

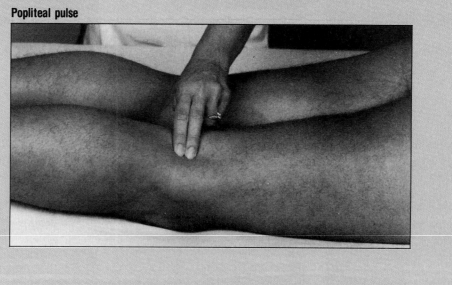

directly reflect the heart's activity.

Once you locate the pulse, check for a regular rhythm. Then, count the beats over 15 seconds, and multiply that sum by 4 to calculate the pulse rate per minute. If the rhythm is irregular, count the pulsations over 60 seconds to determine the rate.

Next, assess the amplitude (or force) of the pulse. Document your findings with a numerical rating from +3 (for a bounding pulse) to 0 (for an unpalpable pulse). Or simply describe the force of the pulse as strong, medium, or weak.

Whenever you encounter an irregularity, auscultate the apical pulse and palpate the radial pulse at the same time. Remember, every time you hear a heartbeat, you should be able to palpate it. If you can't, document the difference between the apical pulse rate and the radial pulse rate. This difference, known as the *pulse deficit*, indirectly evaluates the heart's ability to pump blood to peripheral vessels.

Assessing the patient's respirations

By watching a patient breathe, you can evaluate his lungs' ability to take in oxygen and expel carbon dioxide. Focus especially on the rate, depth, and rhythm of each breath. To determine the respiratory rate (breaths per minute), count the number of respirations over 60 seconds. Do this after taking the pulse and while holding the patient's wrist. In that way, he'll breathe naturally without being conscious of you counting his respirations.

Also judge respiratory depth as the patient's chest rises and falls. Watch for shallow, moderate, or deep breaths, noting the rhythm and symmetry of the chest wall as it expands during inspiration. A normal respiratory pattern is regular, and the patient shouldn't need to use accessory muscles to breathe. Likewise, normal respirations are quiet and easy without abnormal sounds. (See *Identifying respiratory patterns.*)

Identifying respiratory patterns

The rhythm and sound of a patient's breathing create a respiratory pattern that reflects the patient's condition. Common respiratory patterns are identified below.

TYPE	CHARACTERISTICS	PATTERN	POSSIBLE CAUSES
Apnea	Periodic absence of breathing		• Mechanical airway obstruction • Conditions affecting the brain's respiratory center in the lateral medulla oblongata
Apneustic	Prolonged, gasping inspiration, followed by extremely short, inefficient expiration		• Lesions of the respiratory center
Bradypnea	Slow, regular respirations of equal depth		• Normal pattern during sleep • Conditions affecting the respiratory center: tumors, metabolic disorders, respiratory decompensation, use of opiates and alcohol
Cheyne-Stokes	Fast, deep respirations of 30 to 170 seconds punctuated by periods of apnea lasting 20 to 60 seconds		• Increased intracranial pressure, severe congestive heart failure, renal failure, meningitis, drug overdose, cerebral anoxia
Eupnea	Normal rate and rhythm		• Normal respiration
Kussmaul's	Fast (over 20 breaths/minute), deep (resembling sighs), labored respirations without pause		• Renal failure or metabolic acidosis, particularly diabetic ketoacidosis
Tachypnea	Rapid respirations. Rate rises with body temperature—about four breaths/minute for every degree Fahrenheit above normal		• Pneumonia, compensatory respiratory alkalosis, respiratory insufficiency, lesions of the respiratory center, and salicylate poisoning

Measuring blood pressure: Types of equipment

Instruments for measuring blood pressure come in several sizes and styles. For daily use, most hospitals provide an aneroid or a mercury sphygmomanometer and a stethoscope.

For frequent blood pressure readings, the hospital may provide an electronic vital signs monitor. This instrument automatically computes and digitally records the patient's blood pressure. (When using this monitor, remember to manually check the patient's blood pressure on the arm that will be monitored. Then, to confirm the monitor's accuracy, compare the manual reading with the digital display reading.)

Dinamap electronic vital signs monitor

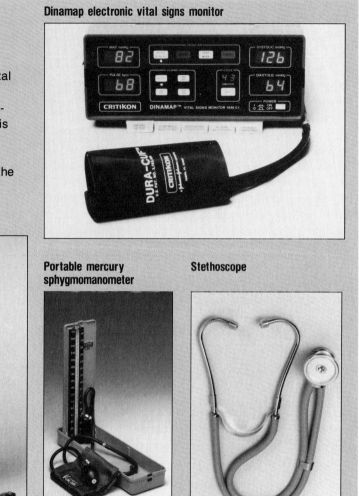

Aneroid sphygmomanometer

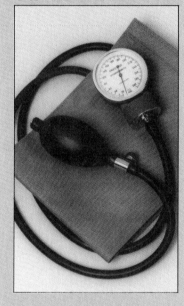

Standing mercury sphygmomanometer

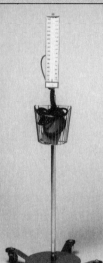

Portable mercury sphygmomanometer

Stethoscope

Taking the patient's blood pressure

When you assess blood pressure, you're indirectly measuring the pressure exerted on the arterial walls with each cardiac contraction. Knowing the amount of this pressure helps you to evaluate cardiac output, fluid volume, circulatory status, arterial resistance, and overall cardiovascular health.

A complete blood pressure measurement reflects the maximum pressure on the arterial wall at the peak of left ventricular contraction (systolic value) and the minimum pressure during left ventricular relaxation (diastolic value). The diastolic value is more significant because it reflects arterial pressure with the heart at rest.

For most patients, you'll take blood pressure with a mercury or an aneroid sphygmomanometer and a

stethoscope. (See *Measuring blood pressure: Types of equipment.*) And in most patients, you'll check blood pressure at the brachial artery.

To record blood pressure accurately, you need to use a blood pressure cuff that fits the patient securely. Follow these guidelines. Use a:
• small, child-sized cuff (9 × 18 cm, or 3½" × 7") when the upper arm's circumference is under 22 cm (8½")
• regular adult cuff (12 × 23 cm, or 4¾" × 9") when the upper arm's circumference is 22 to 33 cm (8½" to 13")
• large adult cuff (15 × 33 cm, or 6" × 13") when the upper arm's circumference is 33 to 41 cm (13" to 16")
• thigh cuff (18 × 36 cm, or 7" × 14") when the

upper arm's circumference exceeds 41 cm (16″).

Initially, you'll measure pressure in both arms, remembering that a pressure difference of 5 to 10 mm Hg between arms is normal. To begin, have the patient lie supine or sit erect with his arm well supported and resting at heart level. Wrap the deflated blood pressure cuff snugly around the upper arm, placing the lower border of the cuff about 1″ (2.5 cm) above the antecubital space. The center of the cuff's bladder should rest directly over the medial aspect of the arm. Many cuffs have an arrow marking the part of the cuff that should be placed over the brachial artery.

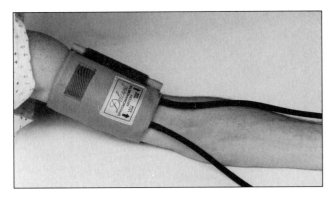

▶ **Clinical tip:** Avoid wrapping the cuff too loosely; this can result in a falsely high reading. Avoid wrapping the cuff too tightly as well; this can result in a falsely low reading.

Palpate the patient's arm to locate the brachial artery; then center the bell of the stethoscope over the part of the artery where you detect the strongest beats. Hold the stethoscope in place with one hand. Using the thumb and index finger of your other hand, turn the thumbscrew on the air pump's rubber bulb clockwise to close the valve.

While auscultating the brachial artery through the stethoscope, pump enough air into the cuff to

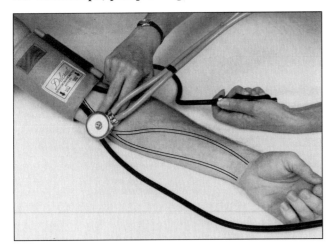

compress and then occlude arterial blood flow. Pump until the mercury column or aneroid gauge registers 160 mm Hg, or at least 10 mm Hg above the level where you auscultated the last sound. Open the air pump's valve, allowing the cuff to deflate slowly (no faster than 5 mm Hg/second). As the air escapes, watch the mercury column (or aneroid gauge) and auscultate the artery. When you hear the first beat or a clear tapping sound, note the pressure on the column (or gauge). This is the systolic pressure (as shown below at left).

The initial beating sound is the first of the five Korotkoff sounds. The second Korotkoff sound resembles a murmur or swish; the third is a crisp, tapping noise; the fourth, a soft, muffled tone. The fifth Korotkoff sound is the last sound heard over the artery.

Continue releasing air gradually while auscultating the artery. When you hear the fifth Korotkoff sound, note the pressure reading. This is the diastolic pressure (as shown below at right).

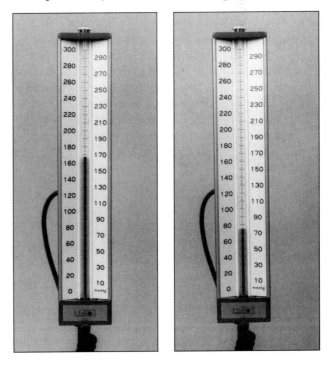

If you continue to hear sounds as the column gauge falls to zero (a phenomenon common in children), record the pressure reading at the beginning of the fourth sound. This is important because in some patients you won't hear a distinct fifth sound.

Now rapidly deflate the cuff and record both pressures. If necessary, repeat the procedure to confirm that your reading is correct. Then remove and fold the cuff and return it to its original storage place.

▶ *Clinical tip:* If you have trouble hearing Korotkoff's sounds, try to intensify them by increasing vascular pressure below the cuff. Palpate the brachial pulse and mark it with an indelible pen. Apply the cuff and have the patient raise his arm above his head.

Then inflate the cuff about 30 mm Hg above his systolic pressure. Lower his arm until the cuff reaches heart level, deflate the cuff, and take a reading.

Alternatively, you can position the patient's arm at heart level, inflate the cuff to 30 mm Hg above his systolic pressure, and ask him to make a fist. Have him rapidly open and close his hand about 10 times before you begin to deflate the cuff and take the reading.

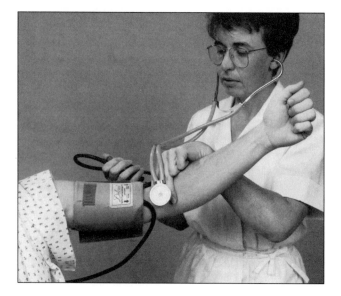

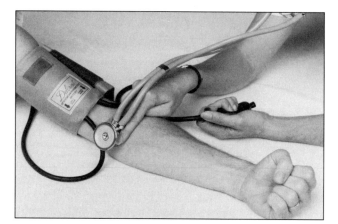

INSIGHTS AND INTERPRETATIONS

Causes of abnormal blood pressure readings

Various factors can cause your patient's blood pressure to rise or fall. The list below identifies these factors.

Elevated blood pressure
- increased cardiac output
- heightened peripheral vascular resistance
- expanded blood volume
- increased blood viscosity
- diminished arterial elasticity
- emotions, such as fear, stress, and anxiety
- pain
- medications

Decreased blood pressure
- reduced cardiac output
- decreased peripheral vascular resistance
- diminished blood volume
- decreased blood viscosity
- increased arterial elasticity
- orthostatic changes
- medications

Assessing the Body

EXAMINING THE HEAD AND NECK

Typically, you'll assess the head and neck to uncover clues to physical problems in the integumentary, musculoskeletal, cardiovascular, respiratory, and neurologic systems. You'll also learn about the patient's nutritional status and sensory problems.

You'll need a clear understanding of head and neck structures to help you detect abnormalities. (See *Anatomy of the head and neck.*) You'll also need to take a health history that focuses on the patient's specific head or neck problem. (See *Exploring complaints of the head and neck.*)

Once you've taken the health history, you can proceed with the physical examination. You'll inspect, palpate, and percuss the patient's skull, scalp, face, and neck to assess the underlying structures, including the skull bones, superficial temporal and carotid arteries, jugular vein, thyroid gland, and lymph glands.

Anatomy of the head and neck

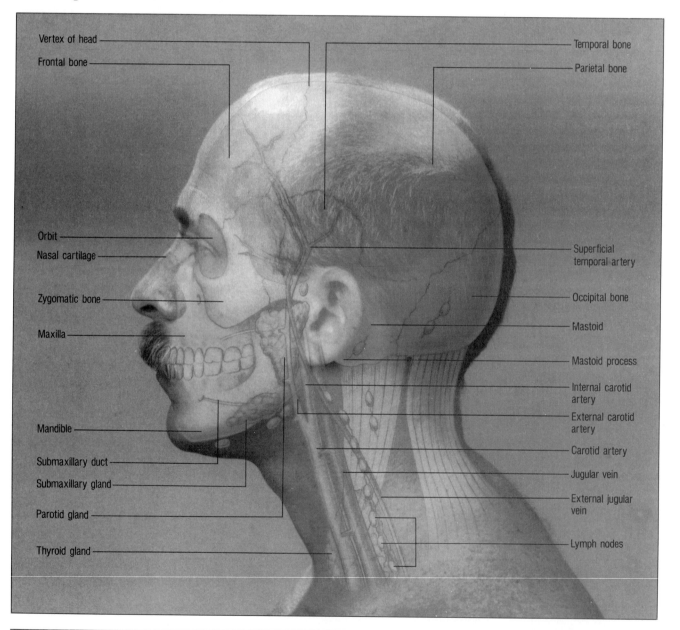

Vertex of head
Frontal bone
Orbit
Nasal cartilage
Zygomatic bone
Maxilla
Mandible
Submaxillary duct
Submaxillary gland
Parotid gland
Thyroid gland

Temporal bone
Parietal bone
Superficial temporal artery
Occipital bone
Mastoid
Mastoid process
Internal carotid artery
External carotid artery
Carotid artery
Jugular vein
External jugular vein
Lymph nodes

ASSESSMENT CHECKLIST

Exploring complaints of the head and neck

To learn as much as possible about a patient's head or neck complaint, focus your assessment on specific problem areas—for example, the patient's medical-surgical history, headaches, mobility, and even the condition of the hair and scalp. Here are some questions to use as a guide.

Medical-surgical history

☐ Have you noticed any lump or growth on your head or neck? If so, when did you first notice it? Has it changed recently? Is it painful?

☐ Have you ever had an operation on your head or neck? If so, when and for what condition?

☐ Have you ever had a problem with your thyroid gland? If so, how was it treated?

Headaches

☐ Do you have headaches? If so, what do you think causes them? How do you relieve the pain?

☐ Do the headaches affect your vision?

☐ Do you ever feel dizzy or faint?

Mobility

☐ Do you have any problems moving your head or neck?

☐ Does moving your head or neck cause you pain? If so, what relieves the pain?

Hair and scalp

☐ Do you have any problems with your scalp, such as itching, dandruff, or sores? If so, has any treatment helped?

☐ Have you changed your shampoo recently?

☐ Have you experienced hair loss? If so, for how long? Is it generalized or localized? Does your family have a history of baldness?

Examining the head

Inspect your patient's head, noting its general size and shape and the skull's contour. Normally, the skull is symmetrical and round. Although skull size varies from one patient to another, a disproportionately large or small skull is abnormal.

Next, palpate the skull. It should feel hard and smooth. Note any deformities, lumps, or areas of tenderness.

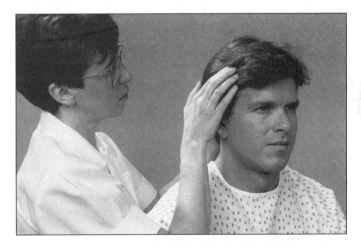

Gently palpate the temporal artery area with your fingertips. Note the character of the pulse, which should be steady.

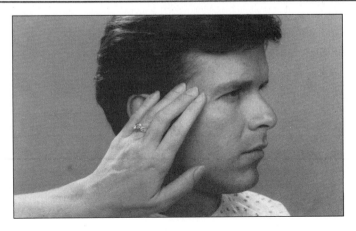

Inspect the patient's hair. Assess thickness, distribution, and texture. Separate the hair into sections with a comb to inspect the scalp. Look for lesions, cuts, scales, and nits.

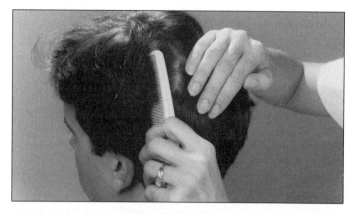

Inspect the patient's face, noting the symmetry of his facial structures. Look for abnormalities, such as drooping eyelids or mouth. Note any involuntary movements, such as facial tics. Inspect the skin for lesions or altered integrity.

   With your fingertips, palpate the facial bones lightly for lumps, tenderness, and edema.

Palpate over the frontal sinuses for tenderness. Press upward from under the bony brow on each side of the face (as shown near right). Avoid pressing on the eyeball.

   Now, using your thumbs, press upward on each maxillary sinus (as shown far right). Note any tenderness.

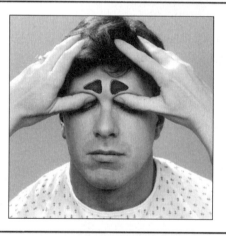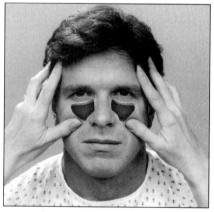

Lightly percuss over the frontal and maxillary sinus areas. Note any tenderness.

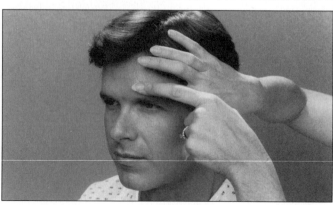

Examining the neck

Working downward, inspect the patient's neck for symmetry and tracheal deviation, jugular vein distention, and carotid artery prominence. Have the patient demonstrate his neck's range of motion by asking him to flex, extend, and rotate his head and touch his ear to his shoulder. Movement should be unrestricted and painless.

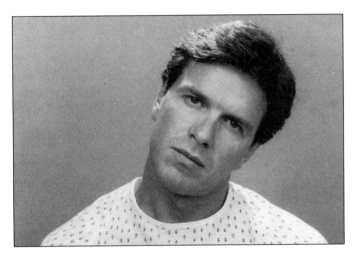

Gently locate and palpate the carotid artery to check the patient's pulse rate and blood flow (as shown near right). Repeat this procedure on the carotid artery on the opposite side. Never palpate both carotid arteries at the same time; this could impede blood flow.

Direct the patient to take a deep breath and hold it. Auscultate over the carotid artery with the bell of the stethoscope, listening for abnormal sounds, such as a bruit (as shown far right). Repeat this procedure on the carotid artery on the other side.

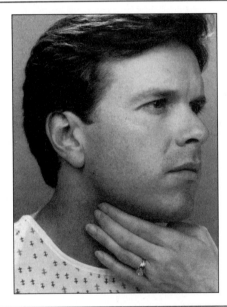

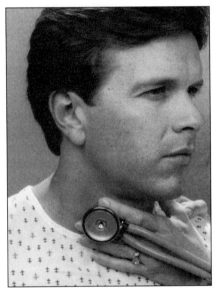

Using the finger pads of both hands, palpate bilaterally under the patient's chin and under and behind the ears. Be alert for lymph node abnormalities. Assess the nodes for size, shape, mobility, hardness, and tenderness.

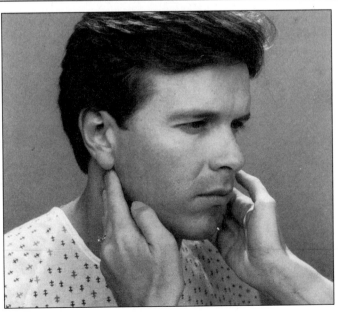

Palpate the trachea, which is normally positioned midline in the neck. Place your thumbs along each side of the trachea near the lower portion of the neck. Determine whether the distance between the trachea's outer edge and the sternocleidomastoid muscle is equal on both sides.

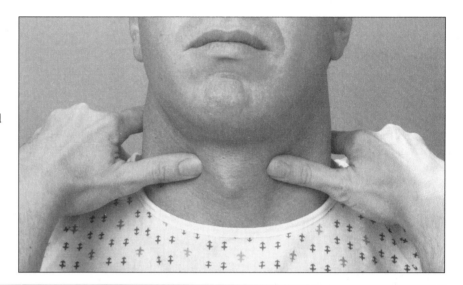

Now feel the thyroid, also to detect deviation or displacement from the midline. Inspect the trachea while the patient swallows. It should move symmetrically during swallowing. Then position yourself behind the patient. Place two fingers from each hand on the sides of the trachea, and ask the patient to swallow. Expect to feel the thyroid move freely.

Displace the thyroid to the right and ask the patient to swallow again. Palpate the right lobe, noting enlargement, nodules, tenderness, or a gritty sensation. Displace the thyroid to the left and palpate the left lobe as the patient swallows.

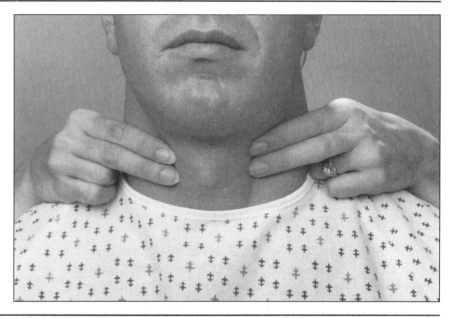

If you detect an enlarged thyroid, auscultate the area with the bell of your stethoscope. Listen for a bruit or a soft, rushing sound indicating a hypermetabolic state.

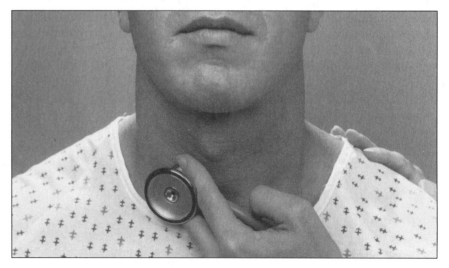

EXAMINING THE NOSE, MOUTH, AND THROAT

No head and neck assessment is complete without a thorough examination of the nose, mouth, and throat. But before you begin your assessment, you'll need to become familiar with the anatomic structures (see *Anatomy of the nose, mouth, and throat*).

You'll also need to take a history of acute or chronic conditions that affect the patient's nose, mouth, and throat. (See *Exploring nose, mouth and throat complaints*, page 25.)

Anatomy of the nose, mouth, and throat

Which structures of the nose, mouth, and throat can provide clues about your patient's condition? Use the following overview as a guide.

Nose

The sensory organ for smell and a filter for the respiratory system, the nose consists of bone in the upper third and cartilage in the lower two-thirds.

Its multifunctional parts are innervated by cranial nerve I, the olfactory nerve. The vestibule (just inside the nostrils) is lined with cilia—tiny hairs that filter inhaled air. The septum separates the nostrils.

(continued)

Lateral view

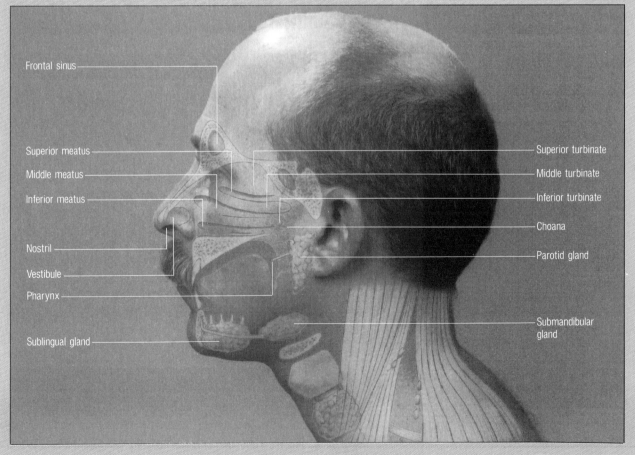

Frontal sinus
Superior meatus
Middle meatus
Inferior meatus
Nostril
Vestibule
Pharynx
Sublingual gland
Superior turbinate
Middle turbinate
Inferior turbinate
Choana
Parotid gland
Submandibular gland

Teresa A. Palmer, RN, MSN, CANP, an assistant clinical professor at the University of Medicine and Dentistry, Newark, N.J., contributed to this section. The publisher also thanks the following for their help: *Melvyn A. Wolf, MD,* Springhouse, Pa.; *Ear, Nose, Throat, and Facial Plastic Associates of Montgomery County, Ltd.,* Springhouse, Pa.; *Hill-Rom,* Batesville, Ind.; and *Hopkins Medical Products,* Baltimore.

Anatomy of the nose, mouth, and throat *(continued)*

Further along the nasal passage are the three turbinates: the superior, middle, and inferior. Separated by grooves called meatuses, the curved bony turbinates and their mucosal covering ease breathing by warming, filtering, and humidifying inhaled air.

Posterior air passages, known as choanae, lead to the oropharynx.

Mouth

The mouth contains the tongue, gums (gingivae), teeth, and salivary glands.

Covered with papillae (small, nipple-shaped projections) that give it a rough surface, the tongue is attached to the floor of the mouth by a frenulum (a restraining band of tissue). The gingivae surround the necks and roots of the teeth, and the mouth's anterior and posterior pillars form a throat cavity that houses the tonsils.

The mouth contains various glands. Three pairs of salivary glands—the parotid, sublingual, and sub-mandibular—secrete into the mouth. The parotid glands are located just in front of and below the external ear; their openings, known as Stensen's ducts, lie in the buccal membrane near the second upper molar. The sublingual glands lie in the mouth under the tongue and open into the mouth floor, posterior to the openings of Wharton's ducts where the mucosa rises to cover them. The submandibular glands lie below and in front of the parotid glands. Wharton's ducts, the openings for the submandibular glands, open onto the mouth floor on either side of the frenulum of the lower lip.

Throat

Located beyond the uvula in a cavity of the oropharynx, the tonsils lie in the throat on both sides of the pharynx. The nearby posterior pharyngeal walls should appear pink, smooth, and dotted with blood vessels and lymphatic tissue.

Anterior view

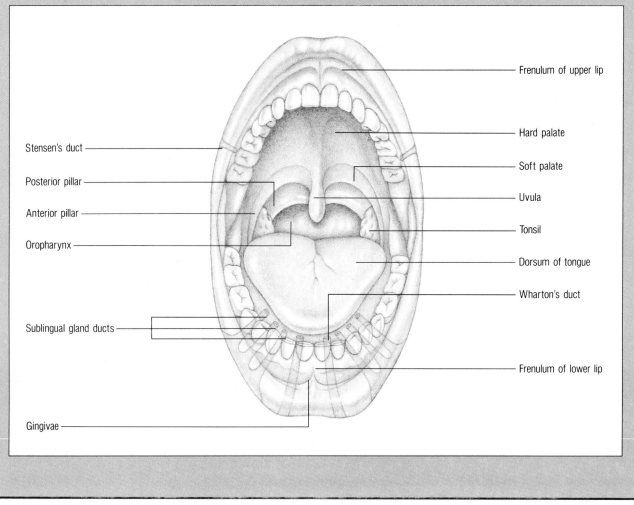

Labels: Stensen's duct, Posterior pillar, Anterior pillar, Oropharynx, Sublingual gland ducts, Gingivae, Frenulum of upper lip, Hard palate, Soft palate, Uvula, Tonsil, Dorsum of tongue, Wharton's duct, Frenulum of lower lip

Exploring nose, mouth, and throat complaints

To investigate your patient's nose, mouth, or throat complaints, ask questions such as these:

Nose

☐ Do you frequently have a runny nose? If so, does it occur at a particular time of year? After specific exposures, such as to pets? In certain environments?

☐ How long do the symptoms last? Are they associated with any other symptoms, such as facial pain and tenderness, headache, or fever?

☐ Do you experience any nasal stuffiness? Does it occur in both nostrils or only one?

☐ Do you ever have a bloody nose for no apparent reason? If so, how severe is it? How often do you have nosebleeds? Do you bruise easily or have bleeding problems in other body areas?

☐ Do you use drugs that you sniff or inhale? If so, what are they? How long have you used them?

Mouth

☐ Do you have bleeding or sore gums?

☐ Do you frequently have ulcers in your mouth or a sore tongue? If so, how frequently?

☐ Do you eat a well-balanced diet?

☐ Do you have any problems with your teeth (such as loose teeth)?

☐ Do you wear dentures?

☐ Do you ever have a "bad taste" in your mouth? When? How often?

☐ Have you noticed any bad breath or other unusual breath odors?

Throat

☐ Do you have frequent sore throats?

☐ Do you have episodes of hoarseness? How long does an episode last? How frequently are you hoarse?

☐ Do you overuse your voice with such activities as singing or yelling?

☐ Do you smoke tobacco or inhale other irritants?

☐ Do you have allergies?

Inspecting the nose

A complete nasal assessment includes the exterior and interior nose. You'll need a good light source, such as a penlight, and a nasal speculum. Don gloves (to protect you from contact with mucus or other body fluids).

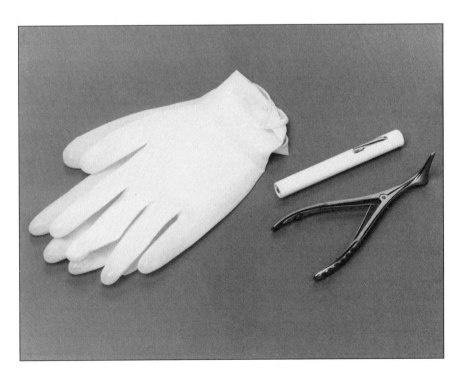

Observe the nose for deviations in its shape, size, or color. The skin should be smooth and lesion-free, and the columella and the tip of the nose should lie midline without deviation. Expect the nostrils to be oval and symmetrical, and watch for nasal flaring or narrowing with respirations—signs of possible airway obstruction. Look for a transverse crease just above the nose's tip—a sign of chronic nasal pruritus and allergies. Note any discharge, and document its character and amount.

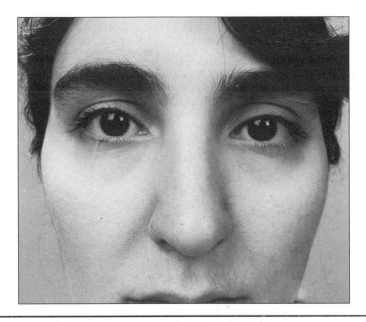

Assess the ridge and the soft tissues of the nose by placing one finger on each side of the nasal arch. Gently palpate, moving the fingers from the nasal bridge to the tip. Note any tenderness or masses.

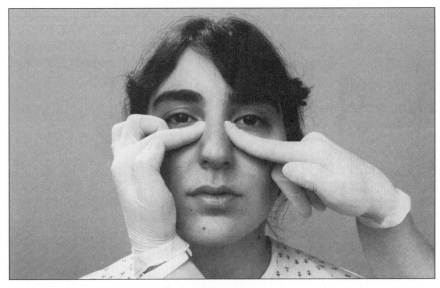

To evaluate patency, occlude one nostril by pressing your finger on the side of the patient's nose. Then ask her to breathe in with her mouth closed. Her breathing should be easy and noiseless. Similarly, check patency on the other side.

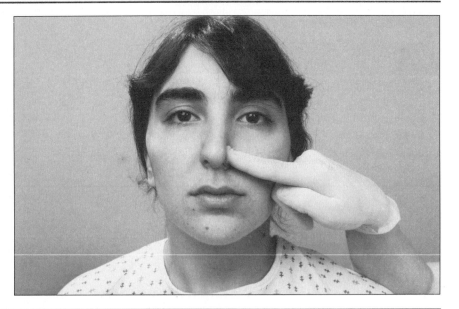

Using a nasal speculum and a good light, such as a penlight, inspect the interior nasal cavity. Hold the speculum in the palm of one hand and the penlight in the other hand. Have the patient tilt her head toward the light source.

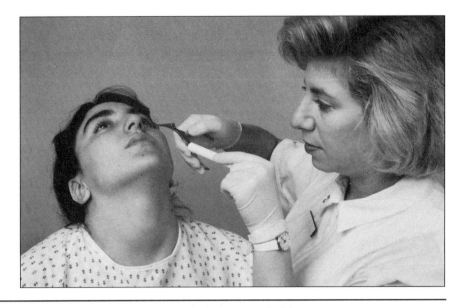

Insert the speculum into the nostril, using your index finger (as shown) for stability. Cautiously open the speculum, being careful not to overdilate the nostril or touch the nasal septum. Inspect the nasal mucosa, which should be deep pink. Note any discharge, masses, lesions, or mucosal swelling. Also check the nasal septum for perforation, bleeding, or crusting. Bluish turbinates suggest allergies. A rounded, elongated projection suggests a polyp.

Next, inspect the opposite nostril. Note any disparity in nostril sizes; such disparity may result from a deviated septum.

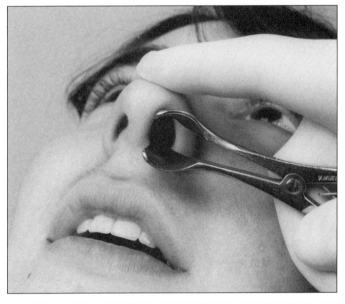

Inspecting the mouth and throat

Before inspecting the mouth and throat, put on gloves. (These are optional, but most nurses wear them.) You'll need a good light source, a tongue blade, and sterile gauze. You may also use a cotton-tipped applicator, if desired, to elicit a gag reflex, although the tongue blade is sufficient.

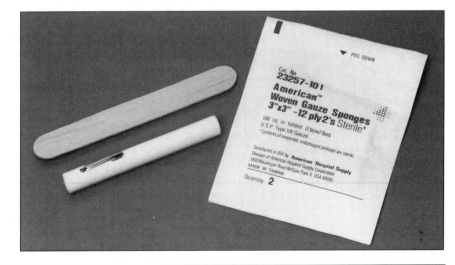

Start by inspecting the lips. Ask the patient to close her mouth, and observe her lips for symmetry and color. Pale lips may reflect anemia; a bluish hue suggests poor oxygenation.

Next, note any edema and alterations in skin integrity. Then palpate for lumps and surface abnormalities (as shown). Dry, split lips may result from dehydration (from wind or heat). Cracks at the corners of the lips may indicate a vitamin deficiency. Edema may result from allergies. Lumps and skin changes may indicate irritation, infection, or cancer.

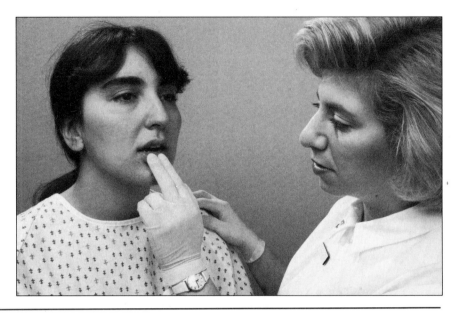

Using the tongue blade and bright light, inspect the oral mucosa. Have the patient open her mouth; then place the tongue blade on the top of her tongue. Inspect the buccal surface of the mouth and lips. Normal mucosa appears moist, pinkish red, and smooth. The gums should appear pink with clearly defined margins at each tooth. Ulcerations, swelling, or bleeding may signal periodontal disease.

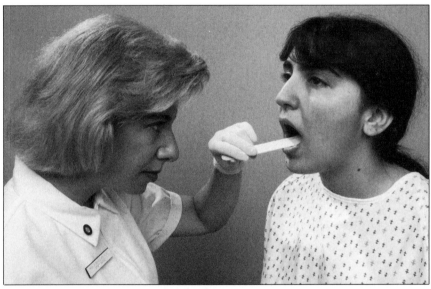

To inspect the dorsum of the tongue, have the patient stick out her tongue as far as possible. A normal tongue appears dull red, moist, and glistening. The anterior surface should be slightly rough with papillae and small fissures. The posterior surface appears smooth and slightly uneven. Look for swelling, color deviations, coating, or ulcerations. Normally, the tongue moves easily. At rest, it should lie straight to the front. Deviation to either side may indicate damage to the hypoglossal nerve.

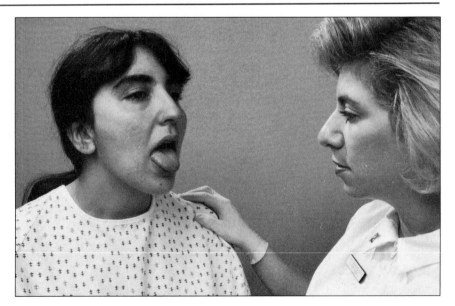

Have the patient place the tip of her tongue on the palate directly behind her front teeth. Inspect the tongue's ventral surface and the floor of the mouth. The ventral surface should be pink and smooth, with large veins between the frenulum and fimbriated folds. Note any swelling and varicosities.

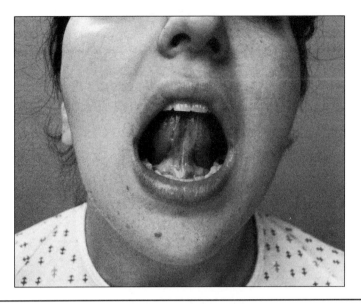

Wrap the tip of the tongue with a piece of gauze. This will help you direct the tongue to one side where you can inspect the lateral borders. Repeat the procedure, and inspect the other side. Both sides of the tongue should have a smooth, even texture. Note any nodules, ulcerations, or white patches.

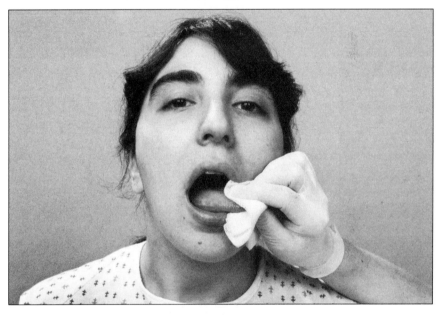

Palpate the tongue and the floor of the mouth, noting any lumps or ulcerations.

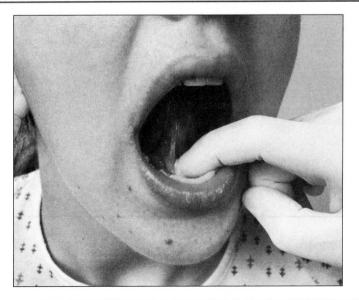

Next, have the patient open her mouth while you shine the penlight on her uvula and palate (as shown). Ask her to tilt back her head, if necessary, to enhance your view. The palate should appear whitish and dome-shaped with transverse rugae in the anterior portion; in the posterior, soft portion, it should appear pink. You may also observe a hard protuberance. At the palate's midline, this protuberance is normal; nodules elsewhere, however, may be tumors.

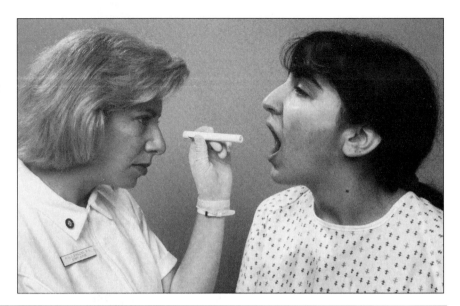

Again using a tongue blade, depress the tongue and have the patient say "ah." Observe the movement of the soft palate and the uvula (lying midline at the back of the soft palate). The soft palate should rise symmetrically with the uvula remaining midline. Deviation to one side may denote paralysis of the vagus nerve.

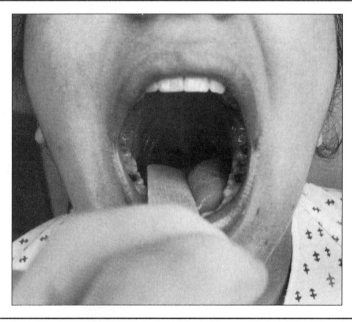

Ask the patient to clench her teeth and smile as widely as possible. The upper teeth should rest evenly on the lower teeth. Note any protrusion of the upper teeth, failure of the upper teeth to overlap the lower teeth, or failure of the upper back teeth to meet the lower teeth (indicating malocclusion). If the patient can't adequately clench her teeth, she may have a damaged facial nerve.

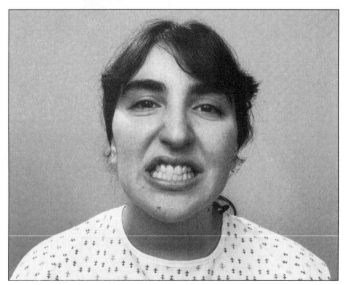

To assess the teeth, have the patient open her mouth wide. Teeth usually appear ivory or slightly yellow although tea, coffee, and tobacco can darken them. Inspect for caries, missing teeth, and loose teeth.

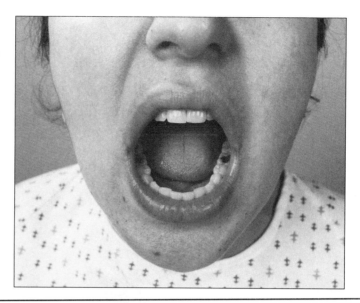

Using a tongue blade, depress the tongue and inspect the pharynx. Note the tonsils on both sides of the pharynx; if they're reddened, swollen, or covered with exudate, they may be infected. Also inspect the throat (pharyngeal) walls. If the tissues appear red and swollen with exudate, suspect infection. If you note yellowish mucoid drainage, suspect allergies.

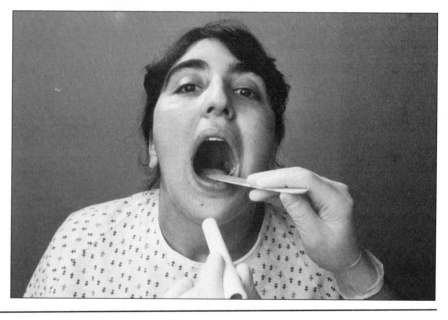

Using a cotton-tipped applicator (or the tongue blade), gently touch the back of the pharynx on each side to elicit a gag reflex. This should produce a bilateral response. Unequal or poor response may signal glossopharyngeal or vagal nerve damage.

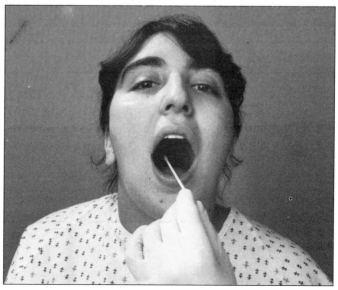

Drug-induced oral and nasal effects

Various drugs can affect the mouth and nose. That's why you must always ask about drug use before concluding that your patient's signs and symptoms result from a disorder. This table lists drugs that may cause oral and nasal effects.

DRUG	ADVERSE EFFECTS
Anticholinergics • atropine, belladonna alkaloids, dicyclomine, glycopyrrolate, hyoscyamine, propantheline, scopolamine	• Decreased salivation, dry mouth
Anticonvulsants • phenytoin	• Gingival hyperplasia
Antidepressants • amitriptyline, desipramine, maprotiline, nortriptyline, trazodone	• Dry mouth
Antihypertensives • clonidine, disopyramide, flavoxate, guanabenz, lithium salts, methyldopa, oxybutynin • guanethidine	• Dry mouth • Dry mouth, nasal stuffiness
Anti-inflammatory drugs • ibuprofen • indomethacin	• Dry mouth, gingival lesions • Gingival lesions
Antineoplastics • bleomycin, chlorambucil, cyclophosphamide, cytarabine, dactinomycin, daunorubicin, doxorubicin, hydroxyurea, melphalan, mitomycin, thioguanine, uracil mustard, vincristine • cisplatin • fluorouracil • methotrexate	• Ulcerated tongue and lips • Gingival platinum line • Epistaxis • Mouth lesions and gingivitis
Antirheumatics • auranofin, gold salts, penicillamine	• Mouth ulcers
Miscellaneous drugs • amphetamines • edrophonium, pyridostigmine • fluorides • isotretinoin • metoclopramide • tetracycline • warfarin	• Dry mouth, continuous chewing or bruxism (grinding) with prolonged use • Increased salivation • Staining or mottling of teeth • Inflamed lips, epistaxis, dry mouth • Dry mouth, glossal edema • Enamel hypoplasia and permanent (yellow-gray to brown) tooth discoloration in children under age 8 and in offspring of pregnant patients • Epistaxis with excessive dosage

EXAMINING THE EYES

Before you can assess your patient's eyes, you need to be familiar with the anatomic structure of this organ. (See *Eye structures and functions.*) Once you're familiar, begin your assessment by asking the patient about any previous eye problems, as well as his present complaint. (See *Exploring eye complaints,* page 35.)

Then, to perform a complete eye assessment, you'll inspect extraocular and intraocular structures and test muscle and nerve function. You'll also investigate visual acuity. Your equipment will include a good light source, one or two opaque cards, an ophthalmoscope, and various vision-test cards. You may also need tissues and cotton-tipped applicators.

Eye structures and functions

During an eye assessment, examine both the eye and related areas. Here's a review of eye structures.
• The white sclera that coats the outside of the eyeball maintains the eye's size and shape.
• The cornea, which replaces the sclera over the pupil and the iris, is a smooth, avascular, transparent tissue that merges with the bulbar conjunctiva at the limbus. Kept moist by tears, the cornea is sensitive to touch (mediated by the ophthalmic branch of cranial nerve V, the trigeminal nerve).
• The iris is a circular contractile disk containing smooth and radial muscles. It's perforated in the center by the pupil. Numerous smooth muscle fibers of varying color make up the iris's surface, giving the eye its color. The posterior portion of the iris con-

tains involuntary dilator and sphincter muscles that control pupil size and regulate the amount of light that enters the eye.
• The pupils should be equal and round. Depending on the patient's age, they may range from 3 to 7 mm in diameter. Infants have small pupils that enlarge during childhood. Pupillary size progressively decreases throughout adulthood and into old age.
• The anterior chamber is filled with a clear, watery fluid called aqueous humor. The fluid drains from the anterior chamber through the canal of Schlemm.
• The lens, located directly behind the iris at the pupillary opening, acts like a camera lens, refracting and focusing the light onto the retina. Composed of

(continued)

Eye structures

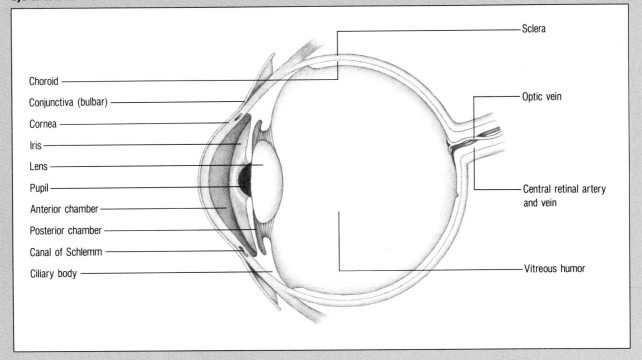

Sclera

Choroid

Conjunctiva (bulbar)

Cornea

Iris

Lens

Pupil

Anterior chamber

Posterior chamber

Canal of Schlemm

Ciliary body

Optic vein

Central retinal artery and vein

Vitreous humor

Eye structures and functions *(continued)*

transparent fibers in an elastic membrane called the lens capsule, the lens contains no blood vessels, nerves, or connective tissue.
• The ciliary body (the thickened part of the vascular coat of the eye that joins the iris and choroid) controls lens thickness and, together with the coordinated action of the muscles in the iris, regulates the light passing through the lens onto the retina.
• The posterior chamber, filled with aqueous humor, is located directly behind the iris, anterior to the lens.
• The vitreous humor consists of thick, gelatinous material and fills the space directly behind the lens. It maintains the retina's placement and the eyeball's spherical shape.
• The posterior sclera, a white, opaque, fibrous layer, covers most of the posterior eyeball. It extends to the dural sheath and covers the optic nerve.
• The choroid, which lines the recessed portion of the eyeball beneath the sclera, contains many small arteries and veins.
• The retina (shown below), the innermost region of the eyeball, receives visual stimuli and transmits the images to the brain for processing. Each of the four sets of retinal vessels, visible through an ophthalmoscope, contains a transparent arteriole and vein. The arterioles are 25% smaller than the veins and brighter in color. As they leave the optic disk, arterioles and veins become progressively thinner, intertwining as they extend to the periphery of the retina.

Each set of vessels supplies a particular retinal quadrant: superonasal, inferonasal, superotemporal, and inferotemporal.
• The optic disk is a well-defined, 1.5-mm round or oval area within the retina's nasal portion. This yellowish orange to creamy pink disk allows the optic nerve to enter the retina at a point called the nerve head. A white-to-gray crescent of scleral tissue may lie on the lateral side of the disk.
• The physiologic cup is a light-colored depression within the optic disk, on the temporal side. The cup covers one-fourth to one-third of the disk but doesn't extend completely to the margin.
• Photoreceptor neurons, called rods and cones, compose the retina's visual receptors. Not visible through an ophthalmoscope, these receptors are responsible for color vision. The rods, concentrated toward the periphery of the retina, respond to low-intensity light and shades of gray; the cones, concentrated in the fovea centralis, respond to bright light and color.
• Located laterally to the optic disk is the macula, which is slightly darker than the rest of the retina and without visible retinal vessels. Because its borders are poorly defined, the macula is difficult to see.
• The fovea centralis, a slight depression in the macular center, appears as a bright reflection in ophthalmoscopic examination. Because the fovea contains the heaviest concentration of cones, it acts as the main vision and color receptor.

Retina

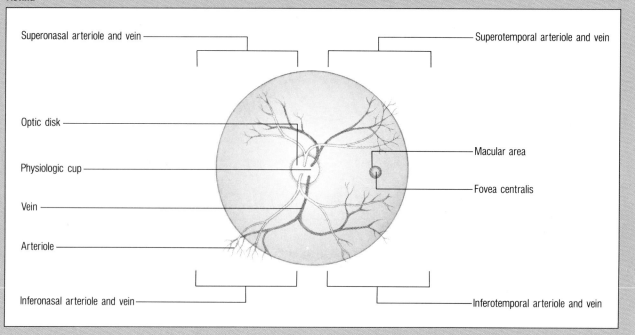

Superonasal arteriole and vein

Superotemporal arteriole and vein

Optic disk

Macular area

Physiologic cup

Fovea centralis

Vein

Arteriole

Inferonasal arteriole and vein

Inferotemporal arteriole and vein

Exploring eye complaints

Use the following questions to elicit information about your patient's eyes.

Vision
- ☐ How do you rate your vision?
- ☐ Do you wear glasses or contact lenses? Do you wear them all the time or just for reading or distance? When did you begin wearing corrective lenses?
- ☐ Have you noticed any change in your vision recently?
- ☐ Do you ever experience blurred vision? Does it become worse at any particular time of the day?
- ☐ Do you have difficulty seeing well at night?
- ☐ Have you ever had double vision? Describe the circumstances.
- ☐ Do you ever see halos around lights? Have you ever noticed blind spots, floaters, or flashing lights? If so, when?
- ☐ Are your eyes unusually sensitive to light?

History
- ☐ When was your most recent eye examination? Were you tested for glaucoma at that time? If not, have you ever been tested for glaucoma? When? Is there a history of glaucoma in your family?
- ☐ Have you ever had a retinal detachment, strabismus, amblyopia, eye injury, or eye surgery?
- ☐ Do you have any eye pain or discomfort? Were you ever treated for eye pain?
- ☐ Do you have allergies? Are they seasonal? Do you know what causes your allergies?
- ☐ Do you have any eye discharge, crusting, or drainage? If so, can you describe it? What color is it? What consistency? Does it have an odor? How long have you had it?
- ☐ Do your eyes tear too much? Too little?

Daily activities
- ☐ Are you exposed to irritating chemicals or gases, foreign bodies, or high-speed machinery at work or home?
- ☐ Do you wear protective eyeglasses during activities that may endanger your eyes?

Examining external eye structures

To assess the external structures, you'll need a penlight, a cotton-tipped applicator, a cotton ball, and an opaque card.

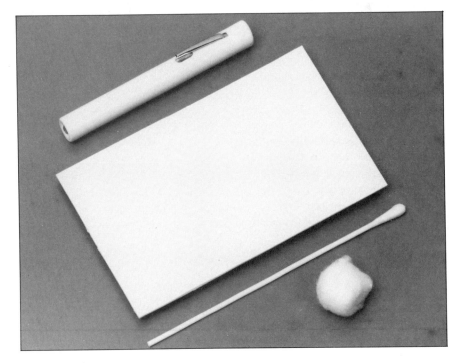

To check the outer eye structures, begin with the eyebrows and look toward the nose. Note any excessive thinning of the eyebrows (a possible sign of hypothyroidism) and altered skin integrity or nits.

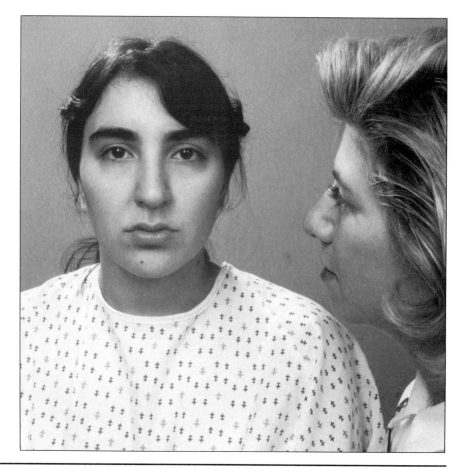

Inspect the eyelids. When open, the upper lid should cover some of the iris but not the pupil. Drooping (ptosis) of one or both eyelids may denote damage to a branch of cranial nerve III. Measure the difference (in millimeters) between the drooping lids, and note any edema, unilateral drooping, or extreme sagging of the lids over the eye.

Eyelid margins should be pink; eyelashes should turn outward. Note any flakiness, redness, swelling, lumps, or suppuration of the eyelid margins. Also observe whether the lower eyelids turn inward toward the eyeball (entropion) or excessively outward (ectropion).

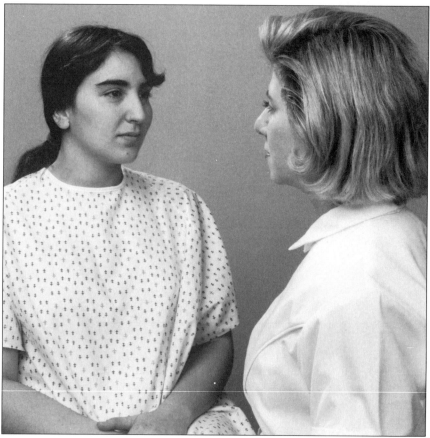

Have the patient close her eyes. Observe for fasciculations or eyelid tremors, possibly indicating hypothyroidism. Be alert for an inability to sufficiently close the lids.

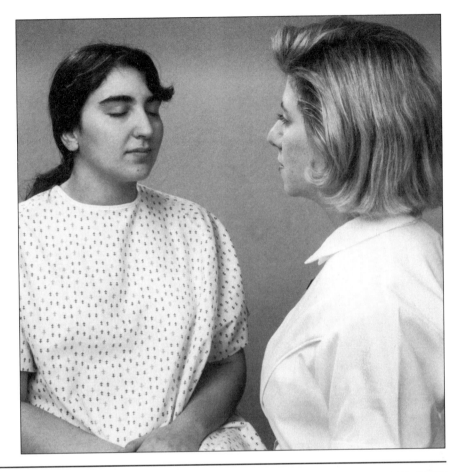

Palpate the eyelids, noting any lumps. Then palpate the eyeball, noting whether it feels excessively hard or whether palpation elicits pain. Hyperthyroidism or a tumor may cause the eyeball to feel resistant upon palpation.

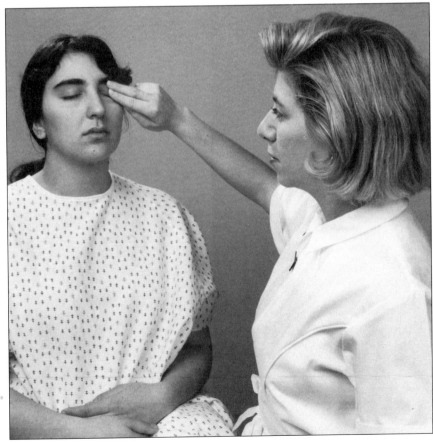

Next, ask the patient to open her eyes and look upward. Place your thumb just under the lower eyelashes and pull down on the lower lid. Inspect the conjunctiva and sclera. Note any excessive redness or exudate. A cobblestone appearance to the conjunctiva on the lid may result from allergies.

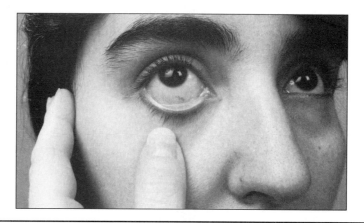

To inspect the conjunctiva and sclera over the iris, place your thumb on the patient's cheekbone and your index finger on her eyebrow. Spread the lids open and tell her to look down.

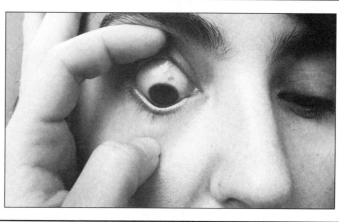

If you suspect a foreign body under the upper lid, place a cotton-tipped applicator on the upper lid just above the eyeball. Have the patient look down. Grasp the lashes on the upper lid and gently pull them down and forward. Using the applicator, gently push down on the upper eyelid and evert the eyelid.

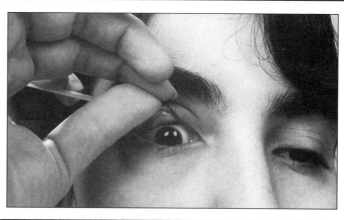

Secure the upper lashes against the eyebrow with your finger and inspect the conjunctiva (as shown). Look for redness, exudate, and foreign bodies. After your inspection, grasp the upper eyelashes and gently pull them forward. Ask the patient to look up. The eyelid should return to its normal position.

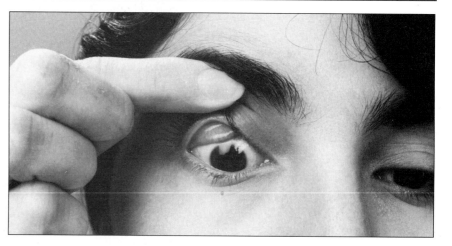

Test corneal sensitivity by touching a wisp of the cotton ball to the cornea. The patient should blink; failure to do so may indicate damage to the sensory fibers of cranial nerve V or to the motor fibers governed by cranial nerve VI. Remember, however, that persons who wear contact lenses may exhibit a reduced response (a result of conditioning to a foreign body).

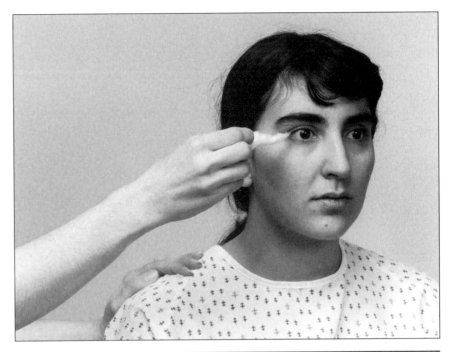

Inspect the pupils. They should be round, regular, and equally sized. Estimate pupil size in millimeters. Unequal pupils, although a normal variant in some patients, generally indicate neurologic damage, iritis, glaucoma, or drug effect.

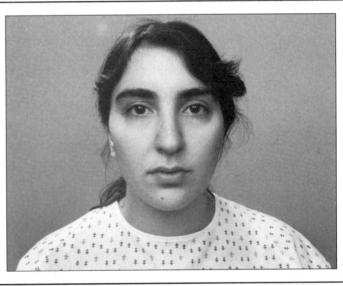

To test the pupils for response to light, dim the lights in the room to allow the pupils to dilate. Shine a penlight directly into one eye and observe pupil constriction. Note whether the other pupil constricts at the same time.

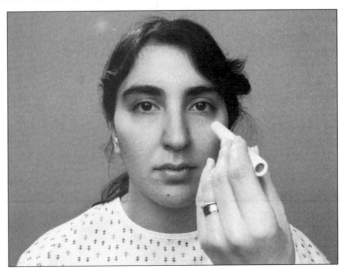

If the pupillary reaction to light appears impaired (or questionable), test accommodation. Hold one finger about 4″ (10 cm) from the bridge of the patient's nose. Ask the patient to look at a distant object and then at your finger. The pupils should constrict when the eyes focus on your finger.

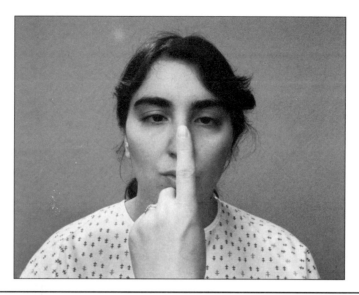

Test the integrated function of cranial nerves III, IV, and VI and the six extraocular muscles by checking the six cardinal fields of gaze. First, hold the patient's chin to prevent her from moving her head. Next, hold one of your fingers up and ask her to watch it as you move it clockwise through the six positions. (Normally, the eyes will move in parallel fashion as they follow your finger.) Then, have the patient look as far as possible to the right. Watch for nystagmus. Finally, have the patient look from the ceiling to the floor and note whether eye movement appears coordinated and smooth.

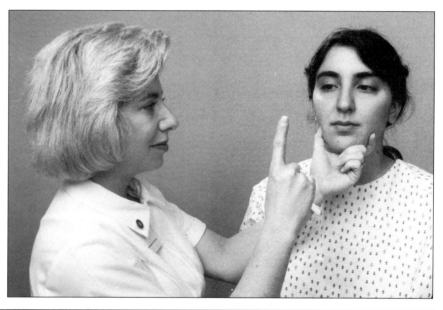

To evaluate the muscle balance that makes binocular vision possible, perform the cover-uncover test. Have the patient stare straight ahead at an object on a distant wall. Cover one eye with an opaque card and observe whether the uncovered eye moves or wanders.

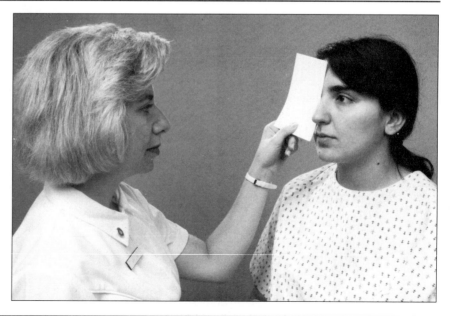

Remove the card from the covered eye; this eye should remain steady, without moving or wandering. Repeat the procedure for the opposite eye.

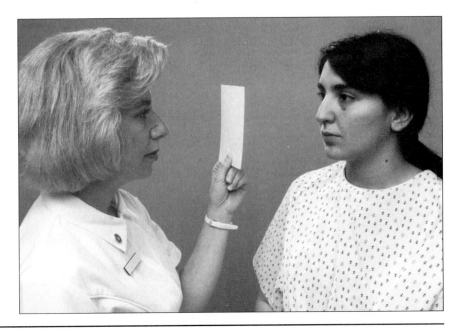

Another test of muscle balance is the corneal light reflex test. Ask the patient to look straight ahead. Shine a penlight on the bridge of her nose from 12″ to 15″ (31 to 38 cm) away. Check to make sure that the cornea reflects the light in exactly the same place in both eyes. An asymmetrical reflex indicates a muscle imbalance. In such a case, one eye is deviated from the fixed point.

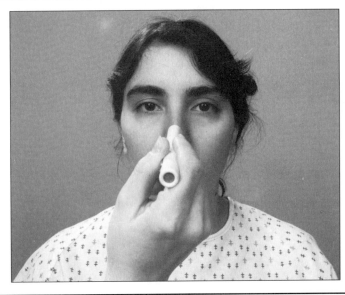

Finally, test convergence. Ask the patient to watch your finger as you move it in from a distance of about 15″ (38 cm) toward the bridge of her nose. Note whether the eyes converge. Normally, the eyes will converge and sustain convergence when your finger is 2″ to 3″ (5 to 8 cm) from the patient's nose. Abnormal or poor convergence may result from hyperthyroidism.

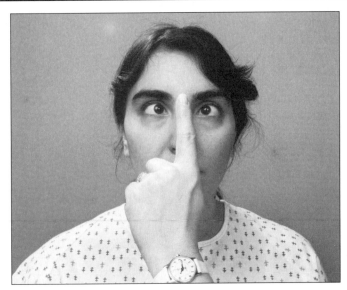

Examining internal eye structures

You'll examine the eye's internal structures with an ophthalmoscope. Made of mirrors, a light, and several lenses, this battery-operated instrument allows you to see such structures as the retina, optic disk, macula, fovea centralis, arteries, and veins.

Front view

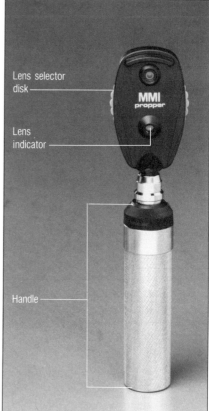

Ophthalmoscope head

Aperture selector

Rheostat

Back view

Lens selector disk

MMI propper

Lens indicator

Handle

Apertures

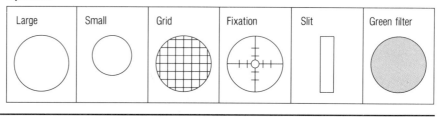

Large	Small	Grid	Fixation	Slit	Green filter

Turn on the ophthalmoscope by pressing the on/off switch and rotating the rheostat clockwise until you reach the desired light intensity. Shine the light onto the palm of your hand, and rotate the aperture selector until a large, round beam of white light appears.

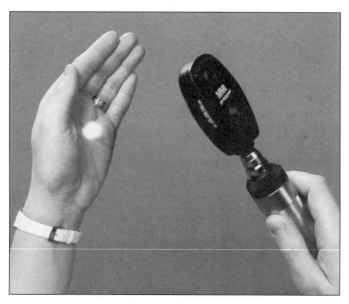

Next, select the proper lens. Choose a lens setting of zero (0) diopter (a measurement of refractive power) if both you and the patient have normal vision. If either of you has myopia (nearsightedness), adjust the lens for a longer focus. Turn the lens selector counterclockwise to the red numbers (negative diopters) until you can see the retina clearly.

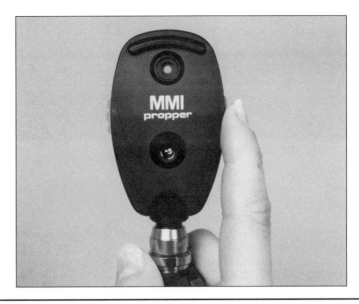

If you need to focus the lens for hyperopia (farsightedness), turn the lens selector clockwise to the black numbers (positive diopters) until you can see the retina clearly. Also adjust the lens to a positive setting if the patient has had a cataract removed, unless this patient wears a contact lens. In such a case, you may be able to see the retina with the lens set at 0.

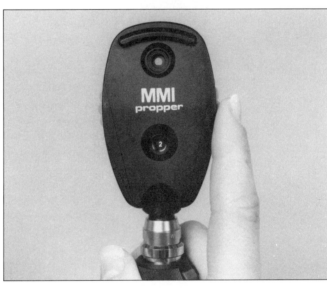

Dim the room lights (to dilate the patient's pupils). If dim light fails to dilate the pupils sufficiently, you may need to administer a mydriatic drug.

▶ *Clinical tip:* Remember, mydriatics are contraindicated for patients with narrow angle glaucoma. They're also contraindicated for patients with head injury or coma who require regular pupillary monitoring.

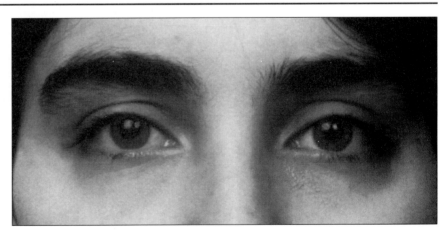

To examine the patient's right eye, hold the ophthalmoscope in your right hand with your index finger on the lens selector so that you can focus during the examination.

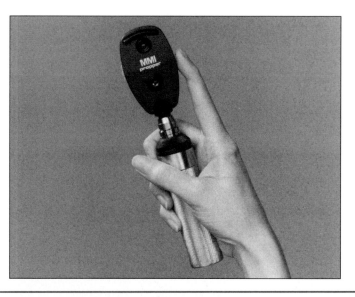

Place the ophthalmoscope over your eye, bracing it near your eyebrow. Make sure you can see through the aperture.

▶ *Clinical tip:* To steady yourself and the patient, place your free hand on the patient's shoulder.

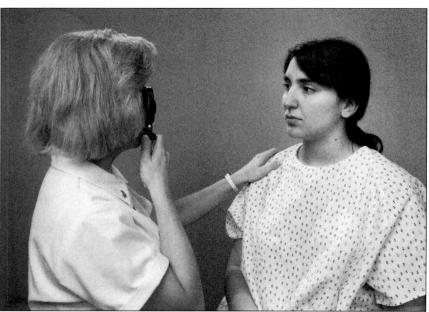

Direct the patient to look slightly up and over your shoulder and gaze at a specific point on the wall. With the ophthalmoscope about 12″ to 15″ (30 to 38 cm) away from the patient, shine the light through the patient's pupil. You'll see an orange glow reflected by the retina. This is called the red reflex. Keeping the light beam focused, move in toward the patient until the ophthalmoscope almost touches the patient's cyclashes.

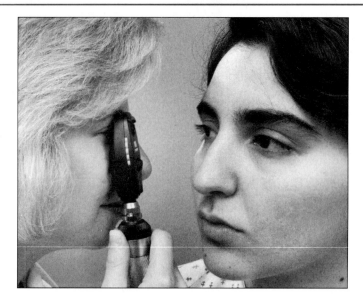

As you approach the patient, retinal details will become sharper although you may need to readjust the lens to keep the retina in focus. If the light shines too brightly, dim it slightly by adjusting the rheostat. Now, look for the optic disk, a yellowish orange to creamy pink oval or round structure located on the nasal side of the retina. If you don't see it, locate a blood vessel and follow it centrally until the optic disk appears.

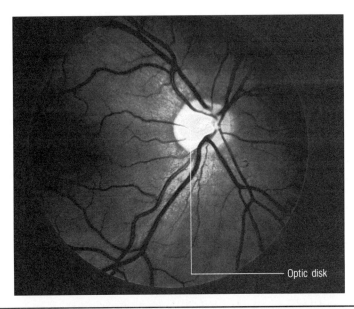

Optic disk

Next, assess the eye's vascular supply by following the vessels in each of four directions. Note the size ratio of arterioles to veins (normally 2:3 or 4:5), and evaluate the character and distribution of the vessels (normally free of exudate) and arteriovenous crossings (normally smooth). As you observe, be alert for lesions.

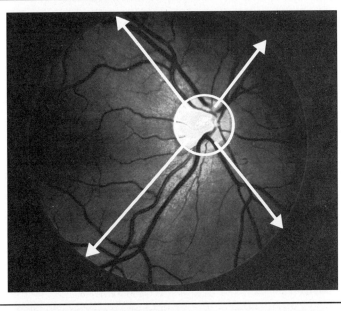

Finally, inspect the macula, located temporally to the optic disk. A normal macula should appear as a yellow dot surrounded by a deep-pink periphery without blood vessels. Repeat the examination on the other eye.

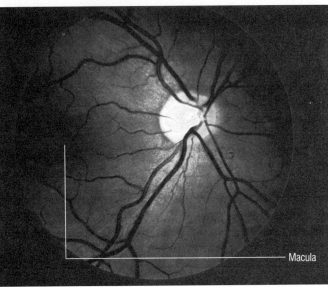

Macula

Testing vision

When you test a patient's vision, you'll examine her far, near, and peripheral vision using a Snellen chart and a near vision chart. Begin by having the patient remove any corrective lenses, if appropriate, and sit or stand 20' (6 m) from the Snellen chart (which should be well lighted). Have the patient cover one eye with an opaque instrument and identify the letters on a line of the chart. (You don't need to start at the line with the largest letters.) Have her read the letters on the next smallest line, and then the next, until she can no longer discern all of the letters on a line. Repeat the test on the other eye.

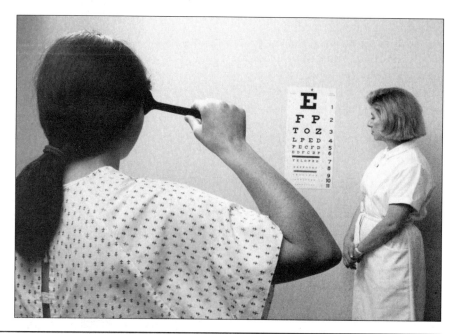

Use the Snellen E chart to test visual acuity in children and other patients who can't read letters. Make sure that the chart is well lighted. Have the patient sit or stand 20' (6 m) from the chart. After covering one of the eyes with an opaque object, point to one of the E's on the chart and ask the patient to indicate the direction in which the letter faces. Repeat the test for the other eye. If the test values between the two eyes differ by two lines, such as 20/30 in one eye and 20/50 in the other, suspect an abnormality such as amblyopia (especially in a child).

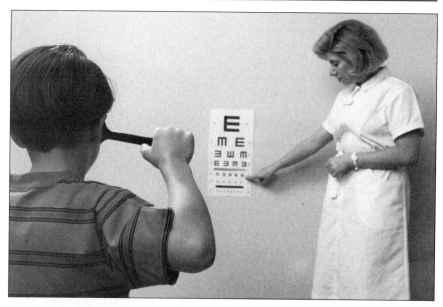

To test near vision, have the patient cover one eye with an opaque instrument and hold a Rosenbaum near vision card 14" (36 cm) from her eyes. Have her read the line that contains the smallest letters that she can discern. Note the measurement indicating near visual acuity. Repeat the test on the other eye. If the patient uses corrective lenses, ask her to wear the lenses and repeat both the far and near vision tests.

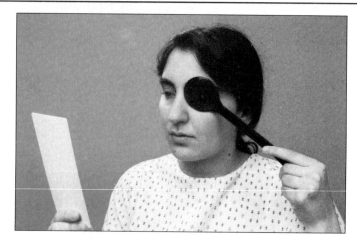

To test peripheral vision, sit about 2′ (61 cm) from the patient and face her. Try to keep your eyes at the same level as hers. Have the patient stare straight ahead. Cover one of your eyes with an opaque instrument or your hand; then ask the patient to cover her eye directly opposite the one you've covered.

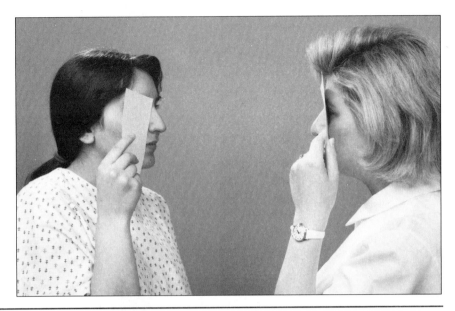

Next, hold up your finger or a pencil at a point equidistant from you and the patient. Move the finger or pencil from the periphery of the superior field toward the center of the field of vision. If you're using your fingers, wave them slightly while moving them in. Ask the patient to tell you the moment that the object appears. If your peripheral vision is intact, the patient should see the object at the same time that you do.

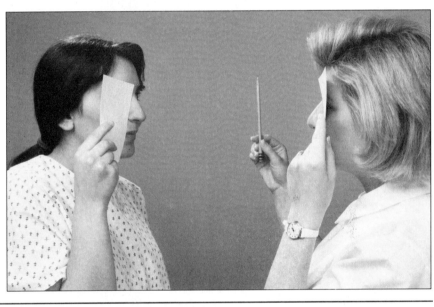

Repeat the procedure in a clockwise rotation to check the inferior, temporal, and nasal visual fields. Then repeat the test on the other eye.

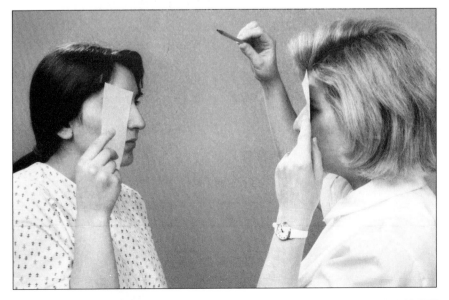

Reviewing common eye charts

You'll use various tools and tests to evaluate your patient's vision. The most commonly used ones include the Snellen charts and the Rosenbaum card.

These devices help you to score the patient's visual acuity. In adults and children age 6 and older, normal vision is measured as 20/20. For children under age 6, normal vision varies: It is 20/50 for children age 3 and under, 20/40 for children age 4, and 20/30 for children age 5.

Snellen charts
You'll use the *Snellen alphabet chart* to detect abnormalities in visual acuity—especially in far vision. The chart has lines of letters in graduated sizes. At the end of each lettered line is a standardized number, which is used to designate the patient's degree of visual acuity when he reads the line from a distance of 20′ (6 m).

You'll record visual acuity as a fraction. The numerator will be 20 (the distance between the patient and the chart); the denominator will be the distance from which a person with normal vision could read the line. The greater the denominator, the poorer the vision.

If the patient can read some but not all of the letters on a line, you'll use that information in the visual acuity fraction. For example, if he can read all of the letters on the line marked 25′, but only two of the letters on the line marked 20′, you'll record the measurement as 20/25 +2. Any measurement less than 20/20 suggests a refractive error or optic disorder.

The *Snellen E chart,* used for children and for adults who cannot read English, records visual acuity in the same way as the Snellen alphabet chart. Instead of various letters, however, this chart includes only E's facing in different directions.

Rosenbaum card
Another common eye chart, the *Rosenbaum card* evaluates near vision. This small, handheld card has a series of numbers, E's, X's, and O's in graduated sizes. You'll hold this card 14″ (36 cm) from the patient and ask him to read the smallest line he can.

Then you'll measure visual acuity by reading the numbers on the right side of the chart. These may be expressed as distance equivalents (such as 20/20) or Jaeger equivalents (such as appear on this card).

Snellen alphabet chart   **Snellen E chart**   **Rosenbaum card**

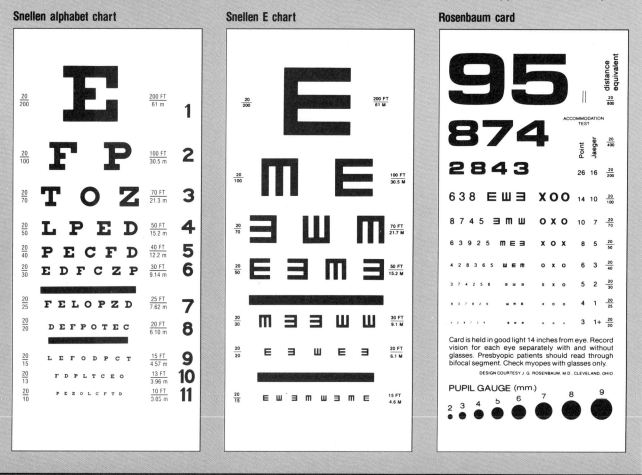

EXAMINING THE EARS

To examine your patient's ears, you need a thorough understanding of this organ's anatomic structures as well as the mechanisms that allow hearing. (See *Ear structures and functions.*)

You also need to recognize typical signs and symptoms of ear problems. The most common ear complaints include earaches, hearing loss, ringing in the ears (tinnitus), and dizziness (vertigo). If the patient complains of ear problems, evaluating his chief complaint can guide your examination and help you determine the cause. See *Exploring ear complaints,* page 51.)

Ear structures and functions

Hearing involves coordination among the ear's three parts (the external, middle, and inner ear) and the cranial nerves. To perform a thorough ear assessment, you need to understand how these structures work.

(continued)

Anterior cross section

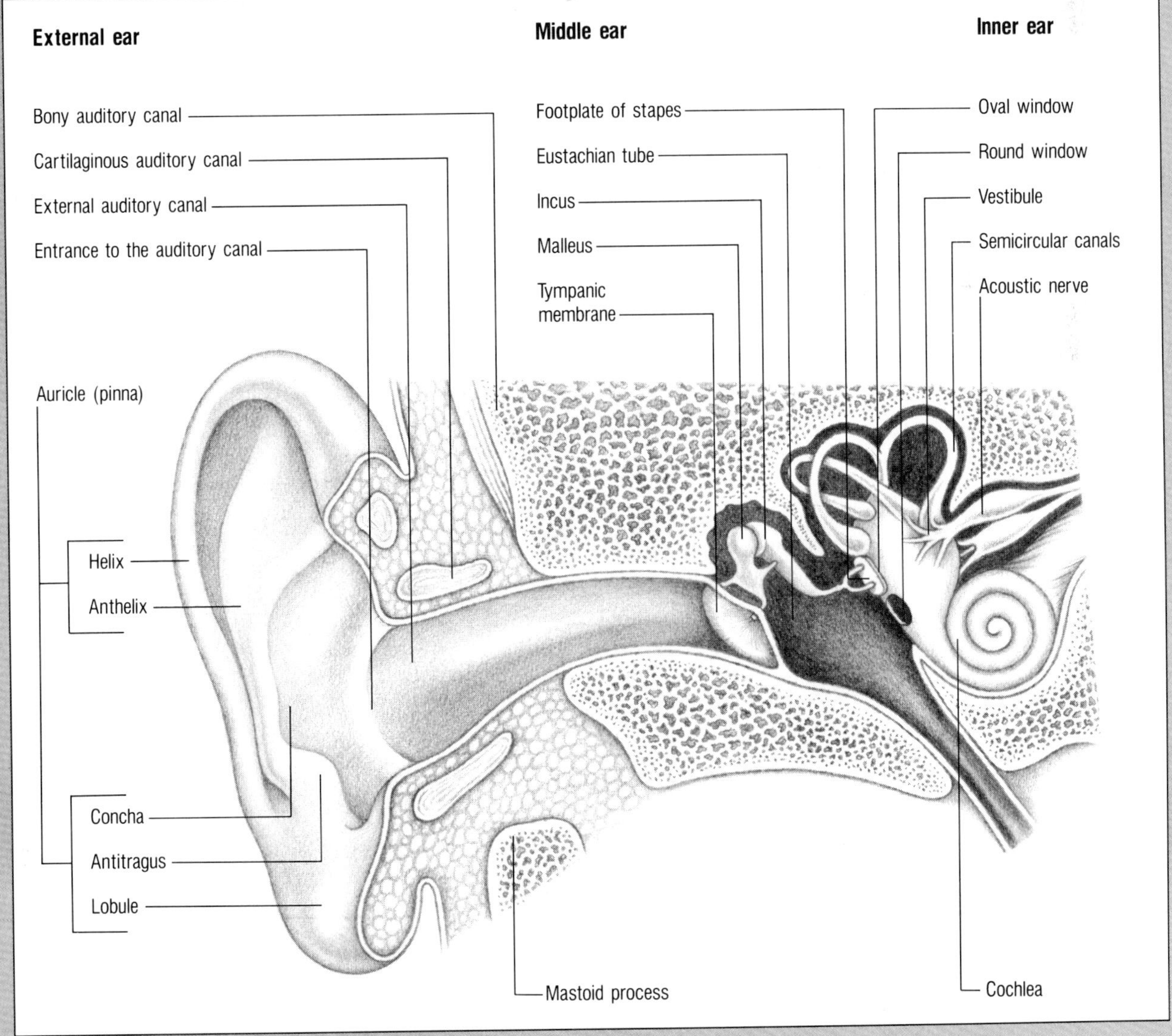

External ear

- Bony auditory canal
- Cartilaginous auditory canal
- External auditory canal
- Entrance to the auditory canal
- Auricle (pinna)
- Helix
- Anthelix
- Concha
- Antitragus
- Lobule

Middle ear

- Footplate of stapes
- Eustachian tube
- Incus
- Malleus
- Tympanic membrane
- Mastoid process

Inner ear

- Oval window
- Round window
- Vestibule
- Semicircular canals
- Acoustic nerve
- Cochlea

Ear structures and functions *(continued)*

External ear

Forming the ear's outer shell are the cartilaginous anthelix, crux of the helix, lobule, antitragus, and concha. Together these parts make up the auricle (pinna). The tragus is anterior to the ear's external opening. Although not part of the external ear, another landmark, the mastoid process, lies posterior to the lower part of the auricle.

Thin, sensitive skin covers both the outer third of the external auditory canal (cartilage) and the inner two-thirds (bone). The adult's external auditory canal leads inward, downward, and forward to the middle ear. The child's auditory canal leads inward, upward, and forward.

Adult's canal

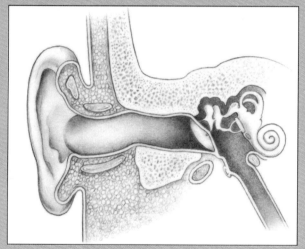

Child's canal

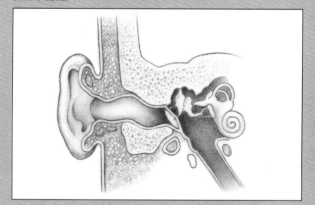

Middle ear

The tympanic membrane (eardrum) separates the middle ear from the external ear. Consisting of layers of skin, fibrous tissue, and mucous membrane, the tympanic membrane is pearly gray, shiny, and translucent. The auditory canal stretches most of the membrane, or pars tensa, tightly inward; a small superior portion, called the pars flaccida, hangs loosely and covers the short process of the malleus. The membrane's center (the umbo) covers the long process of the malleus. Bordering the membrane is a pale, white, fibrous ring (the annulus).

The external canal leads into the middle ear—a small, air-filled cavity in the temporal bone. In this cavity, three small bones, the auditory ossicles—the malleus (hammer), the incus (anvil), and the stapes (stirrup)—link to transmit sound.

During otoscopic examination, you can usually see the handle of the malleus, the short process of the malleus, the umbo, and the cone of light (the light reflex) when you view the tympanic membrane.

The stapes sits in an opening called the oval window. Sound vibrations travel to the inner ear through this window. Covered by a membrane, the round window opens the middle ear to the inner ear. The eustachian tube, which connects the middle ear with the nasopharynx, equalizes pressure between the inner and outer surfaces of the tympanic membrane.

Inner ear

A bony and membranous labyrinth form the inner ear. The bony labyrinth consists of the vestibule, the cochlea, and the semicircular canals. The cochlea contains the organ of Corti for transmitting sound to the cochlear branch of the acoustic nerve (cranial nerve VIII); the semicircular canals contain sensory epithelium for maintaining a sense of position and equilibrium. The vestibular branch of the acoustic nerve contains peripheral nerve fibers that terminate in the epithelium of the semicircular canals, and the central branch terminates in the medulla at the vestibular nucleus.

The hearing pathways

For hearing to occur, sound waves move along two pathways: air and bone. Air conduction occurs when sound waves travel through the external and middle ear to the inner ear. Bone conduction occurs when sound waves travel through bone to the inner ear.

The vibrations transmitted through air and bone stimulate nerve impulses in the inner ear. The cochlear branch of the acoustic nerve transmits these vibrations to the auditory area of the cerebral cortex, where the brain's temporal lobe interprets the sound.

ASSESSMENT CHECKLIST

Exploring ear complaints

If your patient complains of an ear problem, use these questions to guide your history taking. Focus on the patient's past health and his current environment, comfort level, and hearing status.

General concerns

☐ Have you had ear or hearing problems previously? How often?

☐ Do you frequently have ear infections?

☐ Have you ever had ear surgery or been injured on the ear?

☐ Have you recently taken any medications, such as antibiotics? If so, what are they?

☐ How do you perform ear hygiene? Do you insert a cotton-tipped swab or bobby pin into the ear canal?

☐ Do you have a problem with wax accumulating in your ears?

☐ Have you ever had a hearing examination? If so, when? What were the results?

☐ Do you frequently need to ask people to repeat what they've said?

☐ Do you use a hearing aid?

☐ Does anyone in your family have trouble hearing?

Environmental concerns

☐ Do you have any allergies?

☐ Are you sensitive to noise? Are you frequently exposed to loud sound (for example, at work)? Do you often listen to loud music? Do you use a personal radio or stereo cassette with earphones? If so, how high do you keep the volume?

Comfort level

☐ When did you first notice ear discomfort? Did your earache begin suddenly or gradually? How long have you had it?

☐ Where do you have pain? Do you feel it in one or both ears?

☐ Can you describe the pain? Is it constant or intermittent? Do you feel it only when someone touches or pulls your ear?

☐ What, if anything, worsens or relieves the pain?

☐ Do you have any associated symptoms, such as itching or ringing in your ear? Do you feel dizzy? Do your ears feel blocked? Do you have trouble swallowing? Do you have neck or mouth pain?

☐ Have you recently had any problems with your eyes, mouth, teeth, jaws, sinuses, or throat? Did you just have a cold?

☐ Were you recently hit on the ear or were you swimming recently?

Hearing status

If your patient (or his parent) complains of a hearing loss, ask:

☐ When did you first notice a change in hearing? Did it happen suddenly? How long has it lasted? Is the loss constant or intermittent? Did a specific incident precede the hearing loss?

☐ Do you hear better in one ear than the other?

☐ What, if anything, improves or diminishes your hearing?

☐ Do you sometimes shout during a conversation or miss what others say?

☐ Do you (or does your child) often turn up the volume on the radio or television? Does your child tend to ignore you when you speak in conversational tones?

☐ Do voices sound muffled?

☐ Do you ever have ear pain or ringing, hissing, or other unusual sounds in your ears?

If your patient complains of tinnitus, ask:

☐ When did you first notice the abnormal sound? Does it affect one ear or both?

☐ Can you describe the sound? Ringing? Buzzing? Does it sound like air escaping? Is it high-pitched or low-pitched? Constant or intermittent?

☐ Does anything make it better or worse?

☐ Do you have other symptoms, such as vertigo, a hearing loss, or headache?

If your patient reports vertigo, ask:

☐ When did you first notice vertigo? Did it begin suddenly or gradually? Is it constant or intermittent? How long does an episode last?

☐ What were you doing before the first episode occurred?

☐ Did you have vertigo in the past? If so, when? Were the episodes preceded by a special event? How often did they occur and how long did they last?

☐ Do you feel as if you're moving or as if the world is moving around you? Can you walk during an episode or must you sit or lie down? Have you ever fallen during an episode? What, if anything, relieves the vertigo or makes it worse?

☐ Do you have additional symptoms, such as nausea and vomiting or hearing loss?

☐ Do you take any medications? If so, what are they? How often do you take them?

Examining the outer ear

Inspect the auricle of each ear for size, shape, symmetry, color, and position. The skin should be the same color as the facial skin. Observe for moles, cysts, deformities, or altered skin integrity. Also note any drainage from the ear canal.

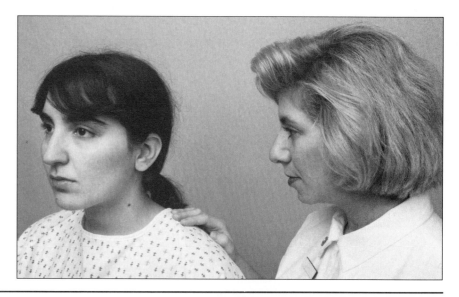

To check the ear's position, draw an imaginary line from the outer canthus of the eye to the protuberance of the occiput. The ear should touch or sit just above this line. Expect the ear to be almost vertical, with no more than a 10-degree posterolateral slant.

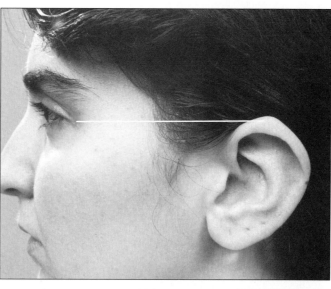

Palpate the auricle (pinna) for tenderness, swelling, or nodules. Gently pull on the tragus and again on the helix to check for pain and tenderness. Gloves are optional for this examination.

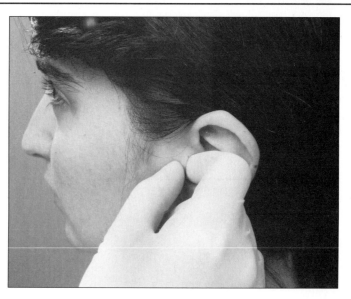

Also palpate the mastoid process. Be alert for pain, tenderness, swelling, nodules, or lesions.

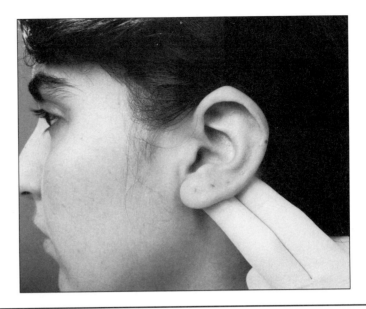

Performing an otoscopic examination

You'll perform an otoscopic examination to see the external ear canal and tympanic membrane directly. To begin, assemble the otoscope (if necessary). Here's how. Attach the handle housing the battery pack to the otoscope's head, which contains a light source and magnifying lens. Select and attach a speculum (lower photograph) large enough to fit the patient's ear canal comfortably. (Speculum sizes typically range from 2 to 9 mm.) Press the light switch on the handle and adjust the beam by turning the rheostat located between the head and the handle. If desired, put on gloves, which are optional for this examination.

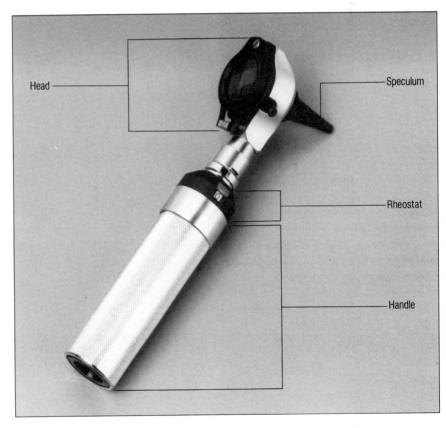

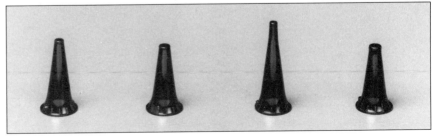

Have the patient sit in a comfortable position or lie down on the side opposite the ear you wish to examine. Hold the otoscope's handle in the space between your thumb and index finger.

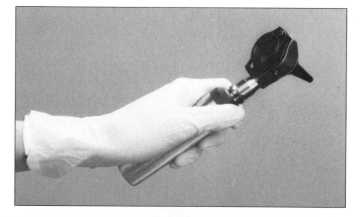

Assist the patient to tilt her head toward the shoulder opposite the ear you're examining. Keeping in mind how the ear canal curves in an adult, gently grasp the auricle and pull it up and back to straighten the ear canal before inserting the speculum.

▶ *Clinical tip:* Keep in mind the sensitivity of the ear canal's skin. Improper technique at this point may cause the patient considerable discomfort or even pain.

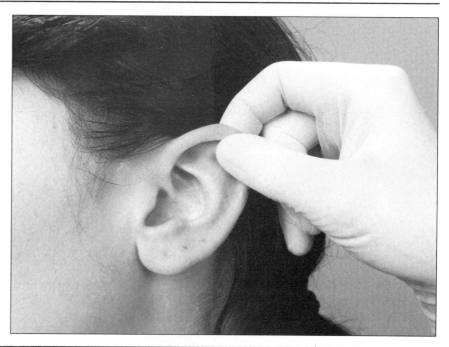

If you're examining a child's ear, pull the auricle gently downward to straighten the ear canal before inserting the speculum.

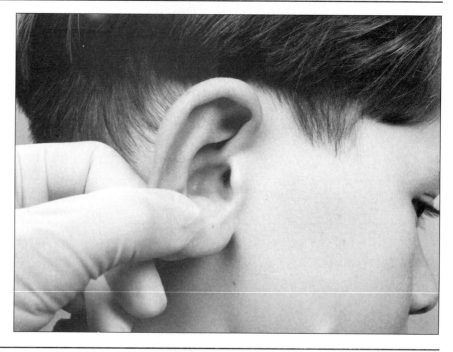

Gently insert the otoscope into the ear canal using one of two techniques: either hold the handle of the otoscope facing down (near right) or facing up (far right). Holding the otoscope with the handle facing up allows you to brace your hand against the patient's head to stabilize the instrument. This helps to prevent injury if the patient moves her head quickly.

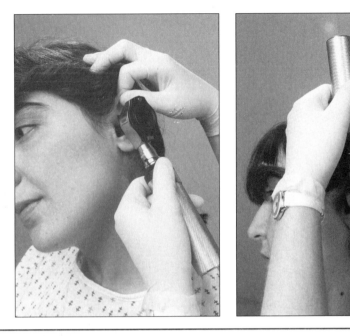

Inspect the auditory canal for cerumen, redness, or swelling. You'll see hairs and cerumen in the ear canal's distal two-thirds. Note excessive cerumen that may obstruct your view; you may need to remove it to complete your inspection.

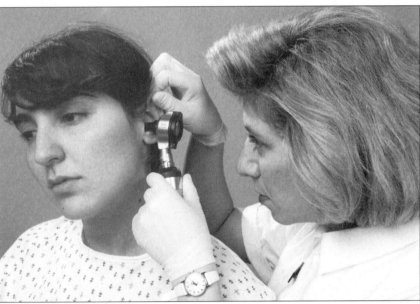

Inspect the tympanic membrane. Typically, middle ear problems will be evident by the tympanic membrane's appearance. Focus on the membrane's color and contour. It should be pearly gray and appear concave at the umbo. Then move the otoscope to identify landmarks on the tympanic membrane, including the umbo, handle of malleus, and cone of light. Be alert for perforations, bulging, missing landmarks, or a distorted cone of light.

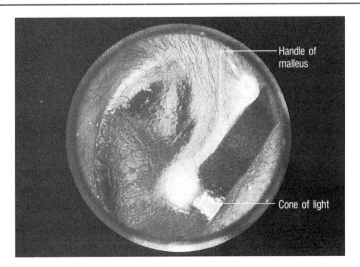

Handle of malleus

Cone of light

Testing hearing

After the otoscopic examination, you'll have an idea of how well the patient hears. If she often asks you what you said or speaks extra loudly, in a monotone, or with erratic volume, you may rightly suspect a hearing problem. To investigate further, use a tuning fork to assess hearing acuity.

▶ *Clinical tip:* Use a tuning fork of at least 512 Hz (or cycles per second), though you may use one that ranges up to 1,024 Hz. These instruments have frequencies that fall within the range of human speech, which is 300 to 3,000 Hz. A tuning fork with a lower frequency—256 Hz, for example—may be better used to assess sensitivity to vibration rather than sound.

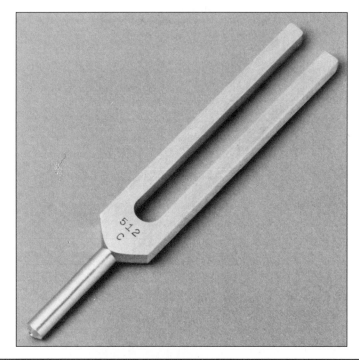

Begin estimating hearing acuity by checking whether the patient can hear you whisper. First, occlude one of the patient's ears by placing your finger in the ear canal. (Gloves are optional.) As you do, gently move your finger up and down. The noise produced will prevent the occluded ear from hearing. This facilitates the assessment of hearing in the other ear.

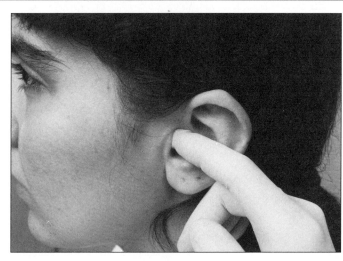

Either cover your mouth or have the patient close her eyes so that she can't read your lips. Standing 1′ to 2′ (31 to 61 cm) away and facing the unoccluded ear, whisper softly and ask the patient to repeat your words. If the patient can't, gradually whisper louder until she can. Use different words each time to ensure that the patient isn't repeating previously uttered words.

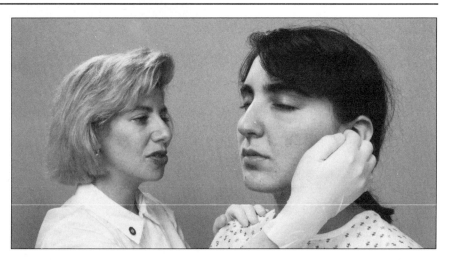

Performing the Rinne test

If you still suspect a hearing loss, perform the Rinne test. This test will help determine whether the loss is conductive or sensorineural. Here's how to proceed. Without touching the tines, hold a tuning fork (either 512 or 1,024 Hz) by its base with one hand. Activate the fork either by stroking it (near right) or tapping it against your knuckle (far right).

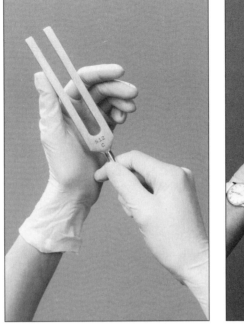
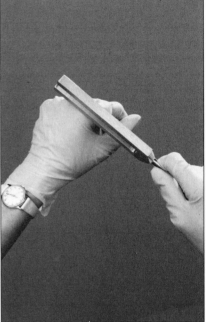

Place the base of the vibrating tuning fork against the patient's mastoid process, and ask the patient to tell you when she no longer hears its sound. Begin timing the interval (counting the number of seconds) until the patient no longer hears the sound.

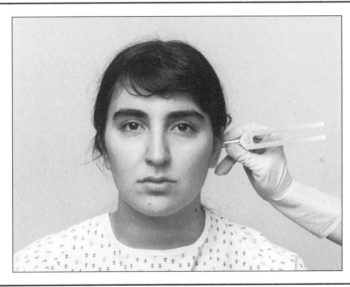

Quickly change the fork's position to about ⅜″ to ¾″ (1 to 2 cm) from the auditory canal. Hold the fork so that the U faces forward, maximizing the sound. Continue timing the interval to determine how long the patient hears this sound by air conduction. Normally, the hearing interval for air-conducted sound should be twice as long as for bone-conducted sound. Repeat the test in the other ear.

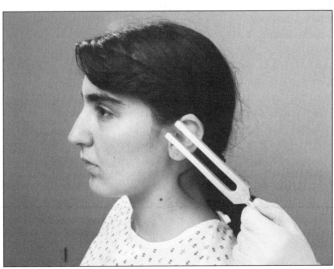

Performing the Weber test

To perform this test, activate the tuning fork as before. Place the base of the fork midline on the patient's head or forehead. Ask whether she hears the sound in one ear or both. Normally, she should hear the sound equally in both ears. If she doesn't, ask her which ear hears better.

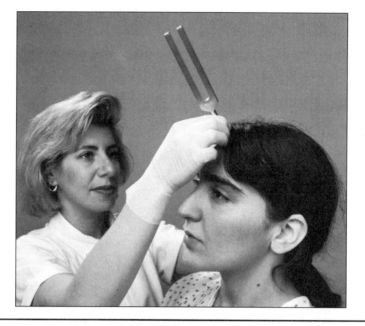

Performing the Schwabach test

To perform this test, occlude one of the patient's ears by gently placing your finger in the ear canal and moving it up and down to block hearing. Activate the tuning fork and place it on the mastoid process behind the opposite ear.

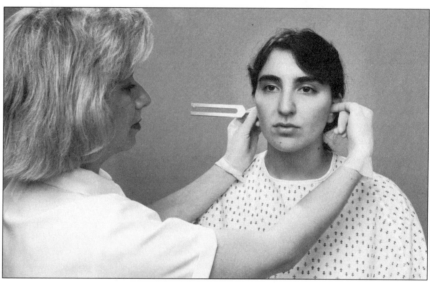

If the patient hears the sound, remove the tuning fork from her mastoid process, occlude one of your own ears, and place the tuning fork behind the mastoid process of your other ear. Alternate the tuning fork between your mastoid process and the patient's, and count the number of seconds until one of you no longer hears the sound. Normally, you and the patient will stop hearing the sound after the same interval.

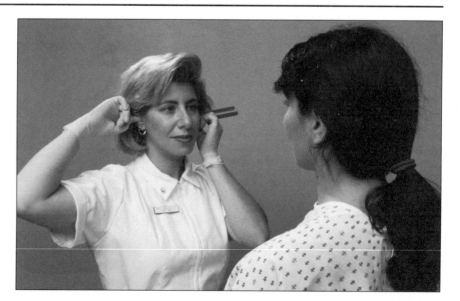

Distinguishing between conductive and sensorineural hearing loss

You use the Rinne, Weber, and Schwabach tests to screen for hearing loss. But you can also use these tests to distinguish a conductive loss from a sensorineural one. This chart explains the test results for each type of hearing loss.

TEST	CONDUCTIVE LOSS	SENSORINEURAL LOSS
Rinne	The patient hears the bone-conducted tone (intensity and volume) as long or longer than the air-conducted tone. Document this result as negative, or − Rinne.	The patient hears the air-conducted tone longer than the bone-conducted tone. Record this result as positive, or + Rinne.
Weber	The patient hears tones louder in the affected ear. Document the result to reflect the ear that hears the louder tones; for example, Weber right or Weber left.	Test results are usually considered inconclusive in this condition. However, you may expect the patient to hear the tone equally or louder in the unaffected ear.
Schwabach	The patient hears the tone longer than the examiner. Document the patient's hearing time in seconds.	The examiner hears the tones longer than the patient. Document the patient's hearing time in seconds.

EXAMINING THE CRANIAL NERVES

During your assessment of the head, neck, nose, throat, eyes, and ears, you evaluated most of the cranial nerves. If you perform a complete assessment of the cranial nerves as you examine the head and neck, you don't need to repeat the specific assessment techniques again.

A summary of cranial nerve assessment techniques and normal findings in adult and infant patients is included here. See *Cranial nerves: Assessment techniques and normal findings*, below, and *Assessing cranial nerves in neonates and infants*, page 62.

Cranial nerves: Assessment techniques and normal findings

The techniques used to assess cranial nerves (CN) vary with the nerve being tested. However, you can assess most cranial nerves when you examine the head, neck, ears, and eyes. The chart below summarizes these techniques and identifies normal findings.

CRANIAL NERVE	ASSESSMENT TECHNIQUE	NORMAL FINDINGS
Olfactory (CN I)	After checking the patency of the patient's nostrils, have him close both eyes. Then occlude one of his nostrils while you hold a familiar, pungent substance—coffee, tobacco, or peppermint—under his nose. Ask him to name the scent. Repeat this test on the other nostril.	The patient can detect and identify the smell. If he detects the smell but can't name it, offer clues such as, "Do you smell lemon, coffee, or peppermint?"
Optic (CN II) and oculomotor (CN III)	To assess the optic nerve, check visual acuity, visual fields, and retinal structures. To assess the oculomotor nerve, check pupillary size, shape, and response to light.	The pupils should be equal, round, and reactive to light. When assessing pupil size, watch for a gradual increase in one pupil or the appearance of unequal pupils in a patient whose pupils were equal.
Oculomotor (CN III), trochlear (CN IV), and abducens (CN VI)	To test the coordinated function of these three nerves, assess them simultaneously by evaluating extraocular movement.	Eye movements should be smooth and coordinated through the six fields of gaze. Observe each eye for rapid oscillation (nystagmus), movement not synchronized with that of the other eye (dysconjugate movement), or inability to move in certain directions (ophthalmoplegia). Also note complaints of diplopia.
Trigeminal (CN V)	• To assess the sensory portion of the trigeminal nerve, ask the patient to close his eyes. Then gently touch the right, then the left side of the patient's forehead with a cotton ball. Ask the patient to signal you immediately when he feels the cotton touch his forehead. Compare his responses on both sides. Repeat the technique on the right and left cheek and on the right and left jaw. Next, repeat the entire procedure using a sharp object. You may use the cap of a disposable ballpoint pen to test his reaction to light touch (dull end) and sharp stimuli (sharp end). (If you observe an abnormal response, test for temperature sensation by touching the patient's skin with test tubes filled with hot and cold water and asking the patient to differentiate between them.) • To assess the trigeminal nerve's motor portion, ask the patient to clench his jaws. Then, palpate the temporal and masseter muscles bilaterally, checking for symmetry. Try to open the patient's clenched jaws. Next, observe the patient open and close his mouth. Be alert for asymmetry. • To assess the corneal reflex, lightly stroke a wisp of cotton across a cornea.	• The patient with a normal trigeminal nerve usually reports feeling both light touch and sharp stimuli in all three areas (forehead, check, and jaw) on both sides of the face. • The jaws clench symmetrically and resist prying forces. • The lids of both eyes will close.

Cranial nerves: Assessment techniques and normal findings (continued)

CRANIAL NERVE	ASSESSMENT TECHNIQUE	NORMAL FINDINGS
Facial (CN VII)	• To test the motor portion of the facial nerve, ask the patient to wrinkle his forehead, raise and lower his eyebrows, smile to show teeth, and puff out his cheeks. With the patient's eyes tightly closed, attempt to open the eyelids. With each of these movements, observe closely for symmetry. • To test the facial nerve's sensory function (taste sensation to the anterior two-thirds of the tongue), prepare four marked, closed containers: one containing salt, a second with sugar, a third holding vinegar, and a fourth with quinine or bitters. Ask the patient to close his eyes while you place salt on the anterior two-thirds of the tongue (with an applicator). Ask the patient to identify the taste as sweet, salty, sour, or bitter. Have the patient rinse his mouth with water; then repeat the procedure. Alternate flavors and tongue sites until the patient tastes all four flavors on both sides. Taste sensations to the posterior third of the tongue are supplied by the glossopharyngeal nerve (CN IX) and usually are tested at the same time.	• Facial movements are symmetrical. • Taste sensations are symmetrical.
Acoustic (CN VIII)	• To assess the acoustic portion of this nerve, test the patient's hearing acuity. • To assess the vestibular portion of this nerve, observe for nystagmus and disturbed balance. Note reports of dizziness or the room spinning.	• The patient hears a whispered voice or a watch tick. • The patient's eyes balance without wavering and he reports no dizziness or vertigo.
Glossopharyngeal (CN IX) and vagus (CN X)	To assess these nerves, which have overlapping functions, first listen to the patient's voice for hoarseness or a nasal quality. Then watch the patient's soft palate when the patient says "ah." Next, test the gag reflex (after informing the patient that you are doing so) by touching the posterior pharyngeal wall with a cotton-tipped applicator or tongue blade.	The patient's voice sounds strong and clear. The soft palate and the uvula rise when the patient says "ah," with the uvula remaining midline. The palatine arches appear symmetrical during movement and at rest. The gag reflex is intact. If the gag reflex appears sluggish or if the pharynx moves asymmetrically, evaluate each side of the posterior pharyngeal wall to confirm integrity of both cranial nerves.
Spinal accessory (CN XI)	To assess, press down on the patient's shoulders while the patient attempts to shrug against this resistance. Note shoulder strength and symmetry while inspecting and palpating the trapezius muscle. Then, apply resistance to the patient's turned head while he attempts to return to a midline position. Note neck strength while inspecting and palpating the sternocleidomastoid muscle. Repeat for the opposite side.	Both shoulders should overcome the resistance equally well. The neck should overcome resistance in both directions.

Hypoglossal (CN XII)	To assess, observe the patient's protruded tongue for any deviation from midline, atrophy, or fasciculations (very fine muscle flickerings that indicate lower motor neuron disease).
	   Next, ask the patient to move his tongue rapidly from side to side with his mouth open; curl the tongue up toward the nose; and then curl the tongue down toward the chin. Use a tongue blade or folded gauze pad to apply resistance to the patient's protruded tongue, and ask him to try to push the tongue blade to one side. Repeat on the other side and note tongue strength.
	   Listen to the patient's speech for the sounds *d, l, n,* and *t,* which require the use of his tongue. If general speech suggests a problem, have the patient repeat a phrase or series of words containing these sounds.
		The tongue is midline and the patient can move it equally to the right and the left and up and down. Normally, pressure exerted by the tongue on the tongue blade is equal on either side. Also, speech is clear.

Assessing cranial nerves in neonates and infants

The techniques for testing a neonate's cranial nerves differ from those for an adult. The chart below summarizes the tests and findings common in neonates and infants.

CRANIAL NERVE	TEST	PROCEDURE	OBSERVATIONS
CN II, III, IV, and VI	Optical blink reflex	Shine a light in the infant's eyes.	• Watch for eye closure and dorsal flexion of head. • The infant will stare intently at a nearby object or examiner's face. • The infant will focus on and track an object with his eyes. • No response may indicate poor light perception.
	Doll's eye maneuver	Same technique as for CN VIII.	• Same response as for CN VIII.
CN V	Rooting reflex	Touch one corner of the infant's mouth.	• Normally, the infant opens his mouth and turns his head toward the stimulus. • Expect little or no response if the infant was fed recently.
	Sucking reflex	Place your finger in the infant's mouth, and feel the sucking action.	• Normally, the infant's tongue pushes up against your finger as he sucks rapidly. • Note the force and pattern of his sucking.
CN VII	Facial expression	Observe the infant when he's crying.	• Usually he can wrinkle his forehead. • Normally his smile is symmetrical.
CN VIII	Acoustic blink reflex	Place your hands about 12″ (30 cm) from the infant's head and clap loudly. Avoid producing an air current with your clap.	• The infant should blink when he hears the sound. • If a neonate or an infant older than 3 days shows no response, he may have a hearing problem. • The infant will habituate to repeated testing. • The infant should move his eyes toward the sound. • When the infant hears a high-pitched sound, he should freeze his position.
	Doll's eye maneuver	Steadily hold the infant under the axilla with him facing you in an upright position. Rotate the infant first in one direction and then in the other.	• The infant's eyes should turn in the direction of the rotation and in the opposite direction when rotation stops. • If his eyes do not move in the expected direction, suspect a vestibular problem or eye muscle paralysis.
CN IX, X, and XII	• Swallowing and gag reflexes • Coordinated sucking and swallowing ability	Pinch the infant's nostrils.	• The infant's mouth will open and the tip of his tongue will rise in a midline position.

EXAMINING THE THORAX AND LUNGS

Typically, you'll assess the thorax and the lungs together because they must work together to sustain respiration. The thorax houses the bones and muscles needed to activate ventilation; the lungs hold the spongy tissues and structures needed for gas exchange. During your assessment, keep in mind that subtle changes in respiratory status may be the first sign of changes in a patient's overall health.

To perform an accurate assessment, you need to understand thoracic and respiratory anatomy and physiology.

UNDERSTANDING THORACIC STRUCTURES

The thoracic cage, which surrounds and protects the trachea, bronchi, and lungs, consists of 12 pairs of ribs, a sternum, and 12 thoracic vertebrae. As a person breathes, the thoracic cage moves constantly, operated by the external intercostal muscles and the diaphragm. The upper seven ribs (also called the "true ribs") connect anteriorly with the sternum; the lower five attach posteriorly to the vertebral column. During assessment, count the ribs and use them as landmarks.

UNDERSTANDING RESPIRATORY STRUCTURES

Air enters the respiratory system through the upper airway, which consists of the nose, nasopharynx, mouth, oropharynx, laryngopharynx, and larynx. The upper airway warms and humidifies the inspired air and acts as the body's first line of defense against infection and foreign bodies. Sneezing, coughing, and gagging allow the body to expel foreign matter.

The lower airway begins at the top of the trachea and includes the bronchi and the lungs, which are responsible for ventilation, perfusion, and diffusion of oxygen and carbon dioxide. They help regulate the body's acid-base balance and form a second line of defense by inducing coughing and bronchial spasms.

At the bottom of the trachea, the bronchi fork into right and left branches (the tracheobronchial tree) and enter the lungs, where they become progressively smaller and divide into the secondary and tertiary bronchi, the bronchioles, and the alveoli.

The right mainstem bronchus is shorter, wider, and more vertically aligned than the left and supplies air to the right lung. This lung is larger than the left, has three lobes, and has a higher percentage of gas exchange. The left bronchus supplies air to the left lung, which has two lobes. The alveolar sacs and the alveoli are the primary areas of gas exchange. (See *Respiratory structures,* page 64.)

UNDERSTANDING RESPIRATORY FUNCTION

Inspiration and expiration result from pressure changes within the lungs. These pressure changes allow the lungs to continually process air—exchanging oxygen and carbon dioxide between the alveoli and the capillaries. This is called diffusion.

Gas exchange and transport

During diffusion, molecules of oxygen and carbon dioxide move between the alveoli and the capillaries. Partial pressure—the pressure exerted by one gas in a mixture of gases—dictates the direction of movement, which is always from an area of greater concentration to one of lesser concentration. In the process, oxygen crosses the alveolar and capillary membranes into the circulatory system, where it dissolves in the plasma and passes through the red blood cell membranes. Here it attaches to hemoglobin, which in turn furnishes body tissues with oxygen. Carbon dioxide moves in an opposite direction—from the tissues, across the alveolar capillaries, and out through the respiratory system.

The circulatory system transports the oxygenated blood from the pulmonary veins to the left side of the heart and then to the rest of the body. The pulmonary arteries transport the deoxygenated blood to the right side of the heart and then into the arterioles and alveoli for exchange in the lungs.

ASKING ABOUT RESPIRATORY HEALTH

Environmental factors, activities of daily living, and family, social, medical, and psychological conditions can significantly affect respiratory function. Consequently, you'll need a thorough history to complement your physical assessment findings (see *Exploring respiratory complaints,* page 65).

Lynne Patzek Miller, RN,C, BS, and *Teresa Palmer, RN, MSN, CANP,* contributed to this section. Ms. Miller is operating room manager at Doylestown (Pa.) Hospital, and Ms. Palmer is an assistant clinical professor at the University of Medicine and Dentistry, New Brunswick, N.J. The publisher thanks *Hill-Rom,* Batesville, Ind., for its help.

Respiratory structures

As you assess your patient, you'll need to keep in mind the underlying respiratory structures, which are shown in the photograph and illustration below.

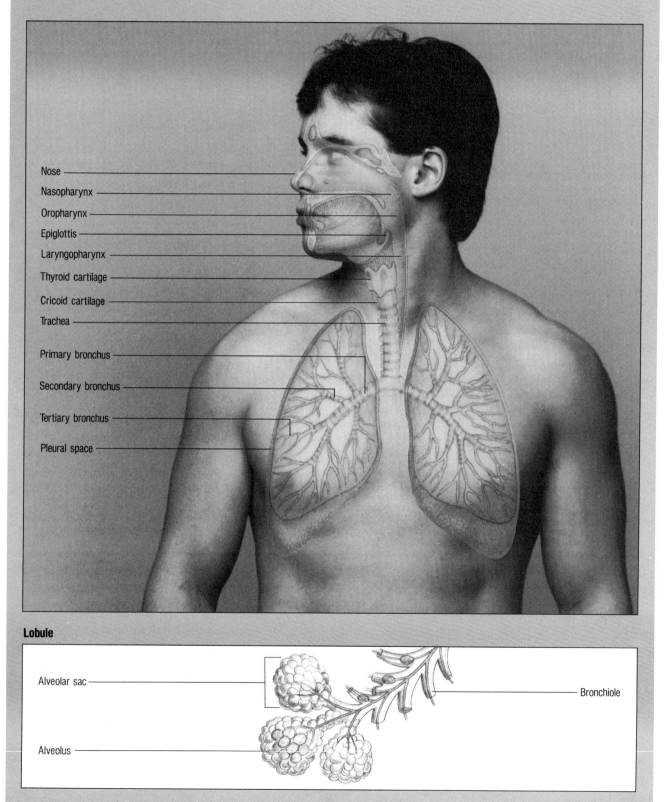

Nose

Nasopharynx

Oropharynx

Epiglottis

Laryngopharynx

Thyroid cartilage

Cricoid cartilage

Trachea

Primary bronchus

Secondary bronchus

Tertiary bronchus

Pleural space

Lobule

Alveolar sac

Bronchiole

Alveolus

ASSESSMENT CHECKLIST

Exploring respiratory complaints

To detect possible abnormalities in thoracic or respiratory status, you'll need to ask the patient relevant questions, such as the ones in this checklist. In addition, be sure to include questions about his health history and activities of daily living.

Thoracic problems
☐ Do you ever have chest pain? If so, point to the exact location. Describe the pain—is it sharp, burning, dull, constant, intermittent?
☐ Can you name or describe any treatments that you received for chest pain?
☐ Have you had a chest injury? If so, when did it occur? Describe what happened.
☐ Can you name the treatment that you received for the chest injury?

Respiratory problems
☐ Have you ever been treated for lung problems? If so, when? What was the lung problem? Describe the details and any treatment that you received.
☐ Do you have a cough? If so, when did it start? Did it begin suddenly or gradually?
☐ Describe your cough—for example, hacking, dry (nonproductive), barking, hoarse, congested, bubbling, or wet (productive).
 Note: Bear in mind that many diseases have characteristic coughs. For example, a congested cough characteristically occurs in pneumonia, bronchitis, and a cold; a dry cough, in congestive heart failure; and a barking cough, in croup.
☐ How often do you cough and for how long? Do you associate coughing with a certain activity, position, or time of day?
☐ Does coughing wake you from sleep? What treatments (prescription or nonprescription drugs, rest, vaporizers) have you tried?
☐ Do you cough up any phlegm, sputum, blood, or mucous plugs?
☐ If so, how much do you cough up?
☐ What color is the substance you cough up? Does it have an odor?
 Note: White or clear sputum results from bronchitis and viral colds, yellow or green sputum from bacterial infections, and pink, frothy sputum from pulmonary edema and pneumonia.
☐ Are you ever short of breath? If so, does this occur suddenly or gradually?
☐ What treatment (medications, change in position, rest) do you use?
☐ Is it harder to inhale or exhale?

 Note: Shortness of breath may indicate musculoskeletal trauma, infection, or such diseases as emphysema, cancer, or heart disease.

Related health history
☐ Do you have any allergies? If so, what kind? Are they related to food, pollen, dust, animals, seasons, or emotions?
☐ Do you have any wheezing associated with your allergies?
☐ What treatments have you received to relieve your allergies?
☐ Do you take any kind of medication—either prescription or nonprescription—regularly?
 Note: Both prescription and nonprescription drugs may cause adverse respiratory reactions, such as dyspnea or respiratory depression. And medications contained in nasal sprays and inhalers may cause a rebound effect.
☐ When was your last chest X-ray and tuberculosis test?
☐ Do members of your immediate family have a history of respiratory disease or allergies—tuberculosis, asthma, or cancer, for example?
☐ Do you have frequent colds?

Activities of daily living
☐ Do you smoke? If so, how long have you smoked, and how many cigarettes or cigars do you smoke each day?
☐ Do you smoke at certain times of the day or during certain activities?
☐ Have you ever tried to quit smoking? If so, what method did you use? Why do you think it didn't work?
☐ Does someone you live with smoke?
☐ Where do you work?
☐ Do you now work, or have you ever worked, in a factory, chemical plant, or coal mine? On a farm? Outdoors in heavy traffic?
 Note: Both primary and secondary smoking can predispose a person to respiratory infections. In addition, air and environmental pollutants can cause respiratory illnesses and deterioration of lung tissue.

Evaluating the thorax and lungs

Begin your assessment by gathering the necessary equipment. You'll need a stethoscope, a marking pen, and a tape measure or ruler. You'll also need an area that's well lighted (preferably with natural light). Typically, your assessment will proceed in this order: inspection, palpation, percussion, and auscultation. You'll finish by assessing respiratory excursion separately.

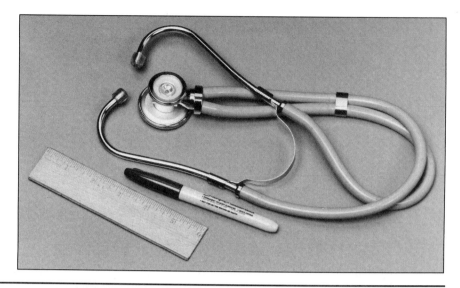

Inspecting the thorax

Help the patient to a sitting position. Then observe his respirations and general appearance. Note his respiratory rate and any unusual breathing pattern. Remember that men and children use the diaphragm to breathe, whereas women use the thoracic muscles. In both male and female patients, be alert for any accessory muscle use.

▶ *Clinical tip:* Watch for use of the sternocleidomastoid, scalene, or trapezius muscles to breathe, or for supraclavicular retractions. If they're present, the patient's inhalation may be impeded. Similarly, watch for prolonged exhalation.

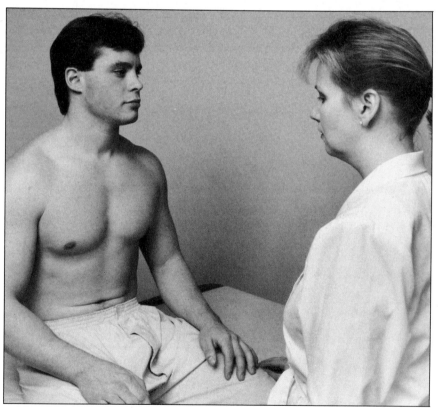

Standing directly in front of the patient, check his skin for discoloration, scars, lumps, dimples, lesions, and ulcerations. Then assess his chest for symmetry, including the symmetry of thoracic and respiratory muscles.

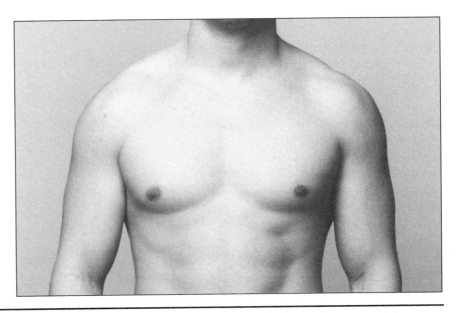

Mentally position the ribs, trachea, and lungs within the patient's anterior thorax.

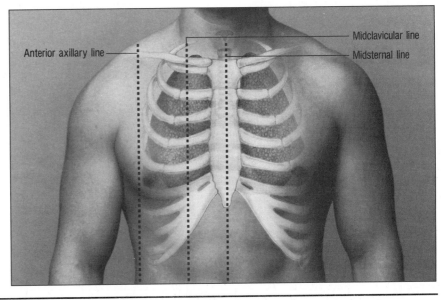

Next, inspect the posterior thorax, noting any skin or other abnormalities. Mentally position the scapulae, ribs, and vertebrae within the posterior thorax.

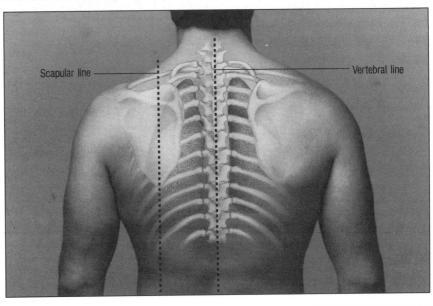

Palpating the thorax

Continue the examination by palpating the patient's thorax. Place the palm of your hand (or hands) lightly on the anterior thorax (near right). Feel for tenderness, alignment, bulging, or retractions of the chest and intercostal spaces. Assess for crepitus, especially around any drainage sites. Repeat this procedure on the posterior thorax (far right).

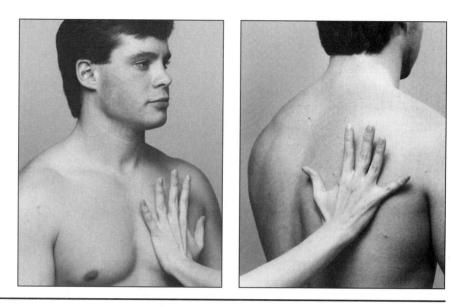

Next, use the pads of your fingers to palpate the anterior and posterior thorax. Pass your fingers over the ribs and over any scars, lumps, lesions, and ulcerations. Note skin temperature, turgor, and moisture. Also note any tenderness or bony or subcutaneous crepitus. The muscles should feel firm and smooth.

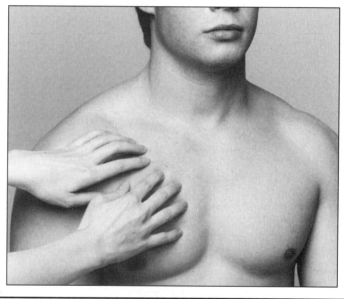

Standing behind the patient, reach over his shoulders and place your hands on his upper anterior thorax, with your thumbs over the sternum and your fingers spreading outward. Ask the patient to take a deep breath and exhale; you should feel the chest wall expand evenly and equally. The patient's shoulders should rise slightly during inspiration and fall slightly during expiration.

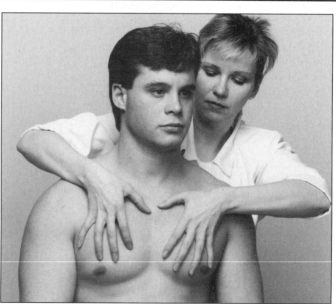

Assess for tactile fremitus by placing your open palms lightly on both sides of the patient's anterior thorax, without touching his chest with your fingers. Ask the patient to repeat the phrase "ninety-nine" loudly enough to produce palpable vibrations. Vibrations that feel more intense on one side indicate tissue consolidation. Less intense vibrations may indicate emphysema, pneumothorax, or pleural effusion. Faint or no vibration in the upper anterior thorax may indicate bronchial obstruction or a fluid-filled pleural space.

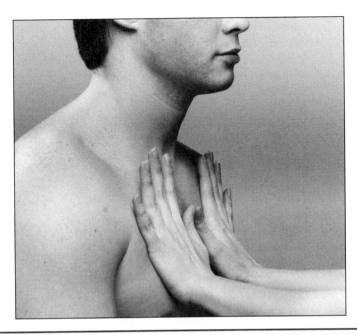

When evaluating the posterior thorax for tactile fremitus, ask the patient to fold his arms across his chest. This moves the scapulae out of the way. Palpate as you would for the anterior thorax.

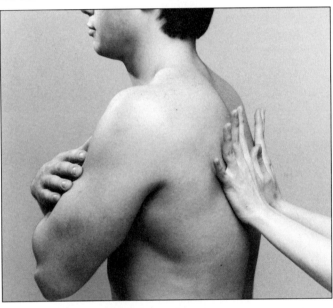

Percussing the thorax and lung fields

Place your nondominant hand on the patient's anterior thorax. Use the tip of the middle finger of your dominant hand to tap on the middle finger of your other hand just below the distal joint. Percuss the patient's anterior thorax at the left clavicle, then at the right.

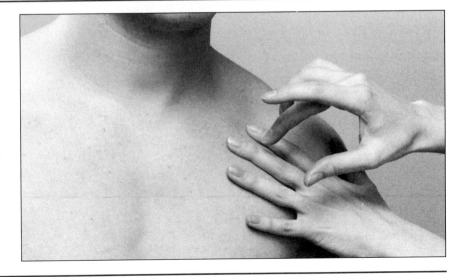

Using uniform pressure, percuss downward and across the anterior thorax (as shown). Note any changes in sound. With *normal* respiratory status, sounds will be low-pitched, moderate to loud, and hollow.

Be alert for these abnormal sounds: *hyperresonance* (low-pitched, loud, longer than normal, and booming) over emphysematous areas and pneumothorax; *tympany* (high-pitched, loud, musical, and drumlike) over a stomach or abdomen distended with air; *dullness* (high-pitched, soft, and thudlike) over solid areas, such as a pleural effusion; and *flatness* (high-pitched, soft, extremely dull, and brief) over areas of atelectasis and extensive pleural effusion.

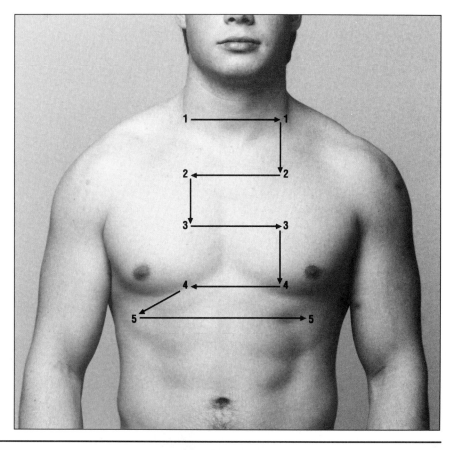

Percuss the patient's posterior thorax, moving downward and across. Note any decrease in sound.

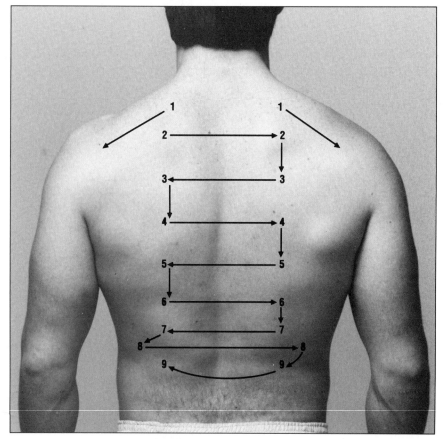

Assess diaphragmatic excursion, or how effectively the diaphragm extends vertically. Begin by asking the patient to exhale. Then percuss to locate the upper edge of the diaphragm (where the normal lung resonance changes to dullness, indicating the position of the diaphragm at full expiration). Mark this spot with a pen.

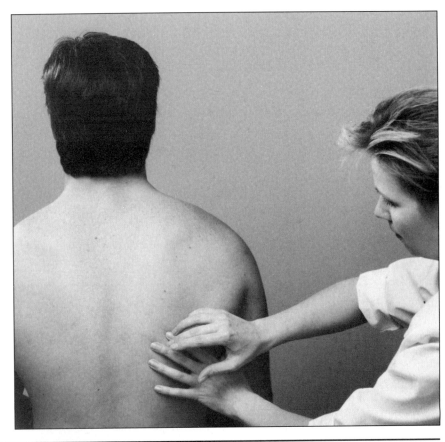

Ask the patient to inhale as deeply as possible. Percuss until you locate the diaphragm at the point of full inspiration. Use the pen to mark this spot as well. Repeat both steps of this procedure on the opposite side of the back.

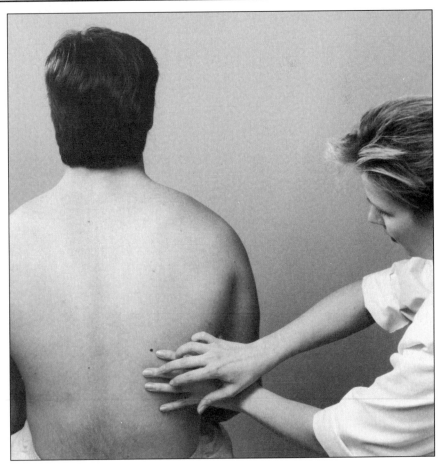

Use a ruler or tape measure to determine the distance between the marks. The distance, which is normally 1¼″ to 2″ (3 to 5 cm) long, should be equal on the right and left sides.

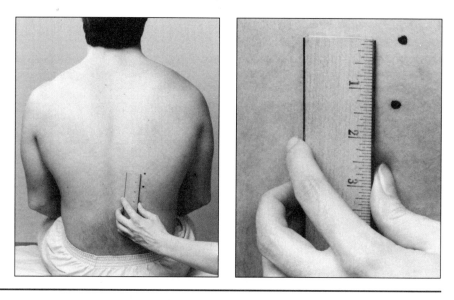

Auscultating the lungs

To auscultate the lungs, ask the patient to sit in an upright position. If he can't sit, have him lie on his side.

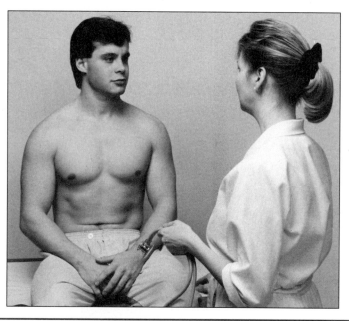

Begin by auscultating the patient's trachea. Continue down over the bronchi between the clavicles and midsternum. When you reach the mainstem bronchus, the sound will be loud, high-pitched, and longer on expiration than on inspiration.

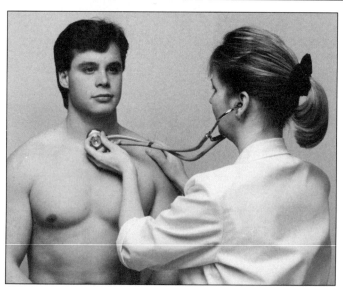

Auscultate the anterior thorax in proper sequence (as shown), assessing for changes in normal breath sounds. Listen for a full inspiratory-expiratory phase at each location. Be alert for crackles, rhonchi, wheezes, and friction rubs, and document their location. Also note any dyspnea, coughing, or chest pain or discomfort that the patient may report.

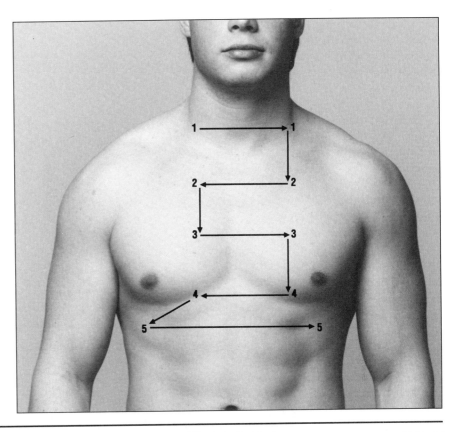

Auscultate the patient's posterior thorax in a systematic right-to-left pattern. Note any abnormal sounds.

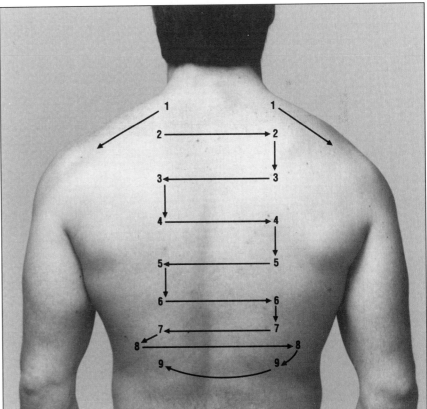

Have the patient say the phrase "ninety-nine." You should hear a muffled, nondistinct sound through the stethoscope. If you hear "ninety-nine" clearly, the patient has bronchophony. Next, have the patient repeat the sound "ee-ee-ee." You should also perceive a muffled, nondistinct sound. If you hear "ay-ay-ay," the patient has egophony. Next, ask the patient to whisper "ninety-nine" while you auscultate. The sound you hear should be barely audible and nondistinct. If you hear "ninety-nine" clearly, the patient has whispered pectoriloquy.

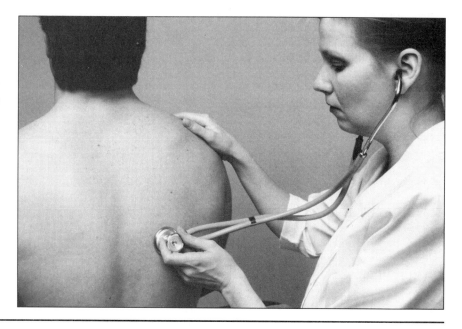

Evaluating respiratory excursion

To assess lung expansion, inspect and palpate three areas on the anterior thorax. Stand in front of the patient. Then place your hands on the anterior thorax at the second intercostal space, with thumbs equidistant from the sternum and fingers spread over the lateral thorax.

▶ *Clinical tip:* To place your thumbs properly, locate the second rib on either side of the sternum. Put your thumbs lightly on the tissue directly below the rib (the second intercostal space).

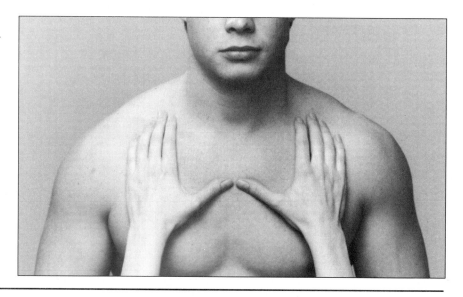

Direct the patient to take a deep breath. As he does so, watch your thumbs move laterally. They should separate simultaneously and equally to a distance several centimeters from the sternum.

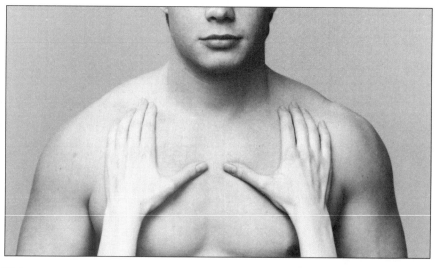

Assess respiratory excursion in the second chest area by placing your thumbs at the fifth intercostal space.

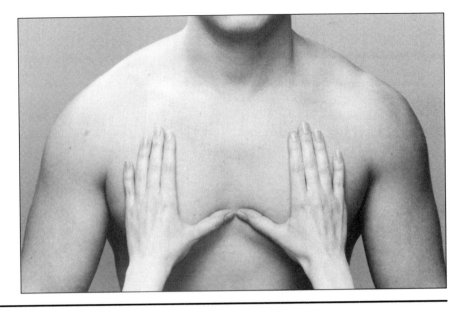

Again direct the patient to inhale, and again watch your thumbs separate. They should move apart symmetrically (as shown). To assess excursion in the third area, position your hands at the sixth intercostal space, and repeat the procedure as before.

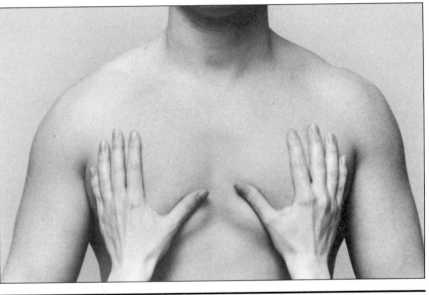

Complete the assessment by inspecting the patient's posterior thorax for respiratory excursion. Stand behind the patient. Position your thumbs so that they touch in the infrascapular area on either side of the spine at the 10th rib. Grasp the lateral rib cage, and rest your palms gently over the posterior surface of the thorax. Avoid applying excessive pressure, which may restrict the patient's breath.

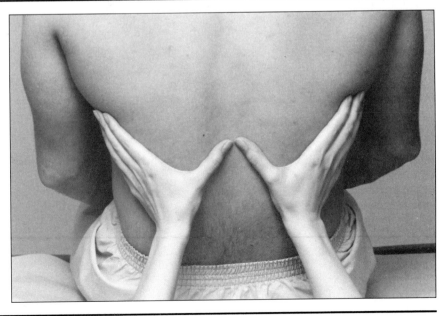

As the patient inhales, expect to see his back move upward and outward and your thumbs move apart (as shown). When the patient exhales, expect your thumbs to return to midline and touch as before. Assess excursion in a second area by putting your thumbs equally lateral to the spine in the infrascapular area, with your fingers extending into the axillary area. As the patient takes a deep breath, expect your thumbs to separate equally as before.

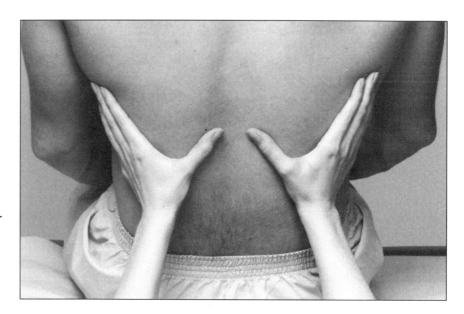

Guide to normal breath sounds

The sound of a patient's breathing indicates the condition of his respiratory and other body systems. To help you assess your patient's breathing, you'll need to recognize normal breath sounds.

Air moving through the tracheobronchial tree normally produces tracheal, bronchial, bronchovesicular, and vesicular breath sounds.

Tracheal and mainstem bronchial breath sounds are heard over the trachea. Loud, high-pitched, and hollow, they're longer on expiration than inspiration.

Vesicular breath sounds are heard over the anterior thorax and the posterior and lateral thorax. They're longer and louder during inspiration than expiration.

Heard over the mainstem bronchi at the first and second intercostal spaces between the scapulae, bronchovesicular breath sounds have a soft, low-pitched, breezy sound. They're lower pitched than bronchial sounds but higher pitched than vesicular sounds.

Anterior thorax

Posterior thorax

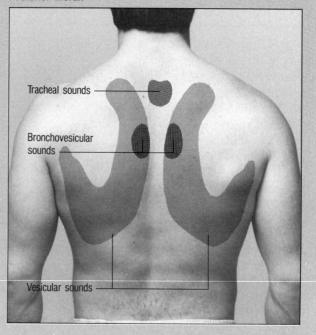

Guide to adventitious breath sounds

Abnormal breath sounds include absent or decreased breath sounds and bronchial breath sounds heard over lung areas other than the mainstem bronchi. Adventitious sounds are also abnormal and may be heard incidental to normal breath sounds. They include crackles, rhonchi, wheezes, and pleural friction rubs. The following information and illustrations will help you recognize the characteristics and location of adventitious sounds.

Crackles

Of the two kinds of crackles, fine crackles can be heard anywhere in the lungs. Typically, you'll first hear them over the lung bases. Their high-pitched, short crackling sounds are heard best on inspiration. Coarse crackles, on the other hand, are loud, low-pitched bubbling and gurgling sounds that start in early inspiration and may last through expiration.

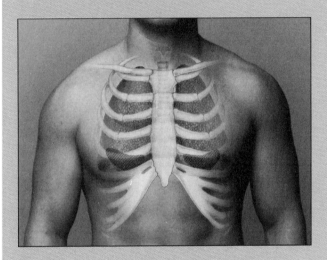

Rhonchi

These abnormal breath sounds are heard over the central airways. They're loud, coarse, low-pitched bubbling sounds heard equally well during inspiration and expiration.

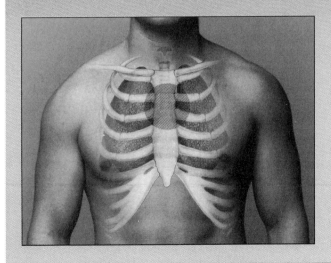

Wheezes

Coming from the large bronchi, wheezes are high-pitched, musical whistling sounds, which may occur during both inspiration and expiration but predominate during expiration.

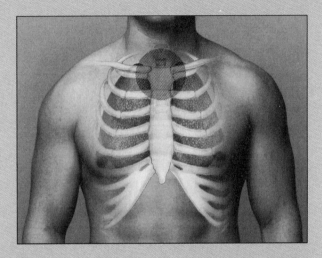

Pleural friction rubs

These coarse, low-pitched abnormal breath sounds are heard at the anterolateral wall during inspiration and expiration.

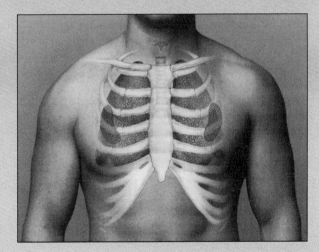

Evaluating respiratory assessment findings

CONDITION	COUGH AND SPUTUM	BREATHING	PALPATION AND PERCUSSION	AUSCULTATION	OTHER FINDINGS
Asthma	• Infrequent cough; nonproductive at first, but increasingly productive as attack worsens • Large amount of tenacious sputum as condition progresses	• Severe dyspnea with prolonged expiration • Intercostal retraction • Possible respiratory arrest	• Decreased or normal tactile fremitus • Increased or decreased resonance	• Decreased breath sounds • Wheezing often audible without a stethoscope and more pronounced on expiration	• Some soreness possible after episode • Extreme anxiety and perspiration
Emphysema	• Chronic hacking cough • Small amount of clear sputum	• Prolonged forced expiration, often through pursed lips • Use of accessory muscles, causing intercostal retraction	• Decreased tactile fremitus • Resonance or (more commonly) hyperresonance • Minimal diaphragm movement	• Decreased or absent breath sounds • Wheezing and rhonchi	• Possible increased anteroposterior diameter (barrel chest)
Pleural effusion	• Occasionally a slight nonproductive cough	• Dyspnea	• Decreased tactile fremitus • Trachea shifted away from affected side • Flat or dull sounds • Decreased diaphragm movement	• Decreased or absent breath sounds over involved area • Egophony and whispered pectoriloquy above fluid level	• Tachycardia
Pneumonia	• Hacking cough; initially nonproductive, but becoming productive and severe as condition progresses • Tenacious and colored sputum (in late stages)	• Increased respiratory rate • Decreased excursion on affected side	• Increased tactile fremitus • Decreased resonance • Decreased diaphragm movement on affected side	• Crackles • Rhonchi	• Sudden, sharp pain in chest area that's aggravated by chest movement • High fever and chills
Pneumothorax	• Nonproductive cough	• Dyspnea • Increased respiratory rate • Cessation of normal chest movement on affected side	• Decreased tactile fremitus • Hyperresonance	• Decreased or absent breath sounds over affected side	• Sudden, sharp pain in chest area • Extreme apprehension, restlessness, drop in blood pressure, and rapid thready pulse

EXAMINING THE HEART

In North America, heart disease represents the leading cause of death and debility. That's one compelling reason for you to make your cardiac assessment thorough and precise. Before beginning, however, make sure that you're familiar with cardiac anatomy and physiology. (See *Cardiac position,* below, and *Cardiac structures and function,* page 80.)

Then assess the patient's history and chief complaints. (See *Exploring cardiac complaints,* page 81). Continue with the examination that appears on the following pages featuring the essential components and techniques of cardiac assessment.

Cardiac position

As you perform a cardiac assessment, keep in mind the heart's location in the chest and its relationship to other organs.

Bony thoracic structures (the sternum and the ribs) protect the heart where it lies obliquely in the chest, with about two-thirds of it located to the left of the sternum. The base of the heart corresponds to the level of the third costal cartilage. Normally, the apex of the heart lies at the fifth left intercostal space, at the midclavicular line. The right end of the inferior surface lies under the sixth or seventh chondrosternal junction. Within the chest, the lungs surround the heart laterally and superiorly. The esophagus lies posterior to the heart; the diaphragm, inferior to it.

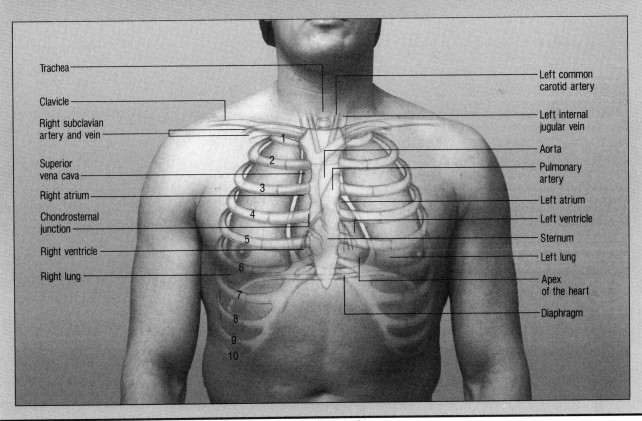

Contributors to this section include *Sandra J. Bixler, RN, MSN, CCRN,* a cardiac clinical nurse specialist at Reading Hospital and Medical Center, Wyomissing, Pa., and *Teresa A. Palmer, RN, MSN, CANP,* a nurse practitioner in adult cardiac surgery at Robert Wood Johnson University Hospital, New Brunswick, N.J. The publisher thanks *Hill-Rom,* Batesville, Ind., for its help.

Cardiac structures and function

As you assess the heart, keep in mind how cardiac anatomy contributes to the heart's central role as a pump, circulating life-sustaining blood to the body's organs and tissues.

Structures
Cardiac structures include the pericardium, three layers of the heart wall, four chambers, and four valves. The pericardium, a closed sac, surrounds the heart and great vessels. The pericardium has an inner (visceral) layer that forms the epicardium and an outer (parietal) layer. The pericardial space between these two layers normally contains from 10 to 20 ml of serous fluid, allowing the epicardium to glide smoothly without friction during heart muscle contraction and relaxation.

The heart wall consists of three layers: endocardium, myocardium, and epicardium. The endocardium (the inner layer) provides a smooth surface for the inner heart structures. The myocardium (the thick middle layer) is made of muscle fibers responsible for contraction. The epicardium forms the thin outermost layer.

The heart chambers include the right and left atria and the right and left ventricles. Heart valves include the atrioventricular (tricuspid and mitral) and the semilunar (pulmonic and aortic) valves. Located at the right atrioventricular orifice, the tricuspid valve consists of three triangular cusps. Located at the left atrioventricular opening, the mitral valve consists of two cusps. Positioned at the orifices of the pulmonary artery and the aorta, the two semilunar valves have three cusps each.

Function
The chambers and valves work together guiding blood through the heart. The arrows in the illustration below indicate the direction of blood flow. The right side of the heart, which includes the right atrium and right ventricle, receives venous blood from the body and pumps it to the lungs for oxygenation. The left side of the heart, which contains the left atrium and left ventricle, receives oxygenated blood from the lungs and pumps it to all body tissues. Blood exits the left ventricle through the aortic valve.

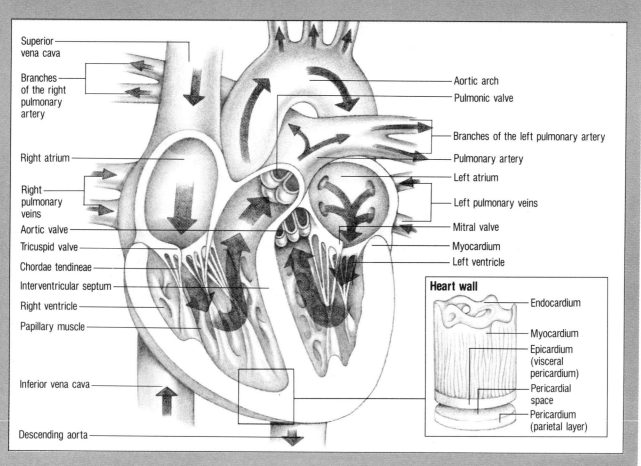

Exploring cardiac complaints

Begin your assessment of the patient's chief complaint by investigating his cardiac health history. Ask the patient why he's seeking medical care. Document his answer in his own words.

If the patient has a medical complaint, ask how long he's had the problem and when it began. Explore any associated signs and symptoms. If he reports chest pain, ask about the pain's location, radiation, intensity, and duration. Also ask about precipitating, exacerbating, and relieving factors. If the patient is experiencing chest pain during the assessment, obtain as accurate a description as possible.

As you interview the patient and compile assessment data, remember to avoid leading questions and to use familiar expressions rather than medical terms. If the patient isn't in distress, ask open-ended questions, which require more than a yes-or-no response. Simultaneously, perform the physical examination, proceeding from inspection and palpation through percussion and auscultation.

Use the following questions to help your patient accurately describe his cardiovascular symptoms.
□ Where in your chest do you feel pain?
□ Can you point to the site of your pain? Does it radiate to any other areas?

□ Do you get a burning or squeezing sensation in your chest?
□ How long have you been having chest pain? How long does an attack last?
□ What relieves the pain?
□ How would you rate the intensity of your pain on a scale of 1 to 10, with 10 as the most severe pain?
□ Do you ever feel short of breath? Does a particular body position seem to bring this on? Which one? How long does any shortness of breath last? What relieves it?
□ Has breathing trouble ever awakened you from sleep?
□ Do you ever wake up coughing? How often?
□ Have you ever coughed up blood?
□ Does your heart ever pound, race, or skip a beat? If so, when does this happen?
□ Do you ever feel dizzy or faint? What seems to bring this on?
□ Do your feet or ankles swell? At what time of day? What, if anything, relieves the swelling?
□ Do you urinate more frequently at night?
□ Do any activities easily tire you? Which ones? Have you had to limit your activities or rest more often while doing them? Does rest relieve the fatigue?

Inspecting the jugular veins

You'll need only your stethoscope, a light source, a centimeter ruler, and a warm, quiet, private setting with adequate lighting. Wash your hands and explain the procedure to the patient. Begin by observing the jugular veins to detect distention. Assist the patient into semi-Fowler's position. Turn his head slightly away from the side you're examining. Angle the light source (a penlight, for example) to cast shadows along the neck. (The shadows will help you see pulse wave motion.) Measure the level of distention in fingerbreadths above the clavicle.

▶ *Clinical tip:* You'll see jugular vein distention only if the patient has right ventricular dysfunction.

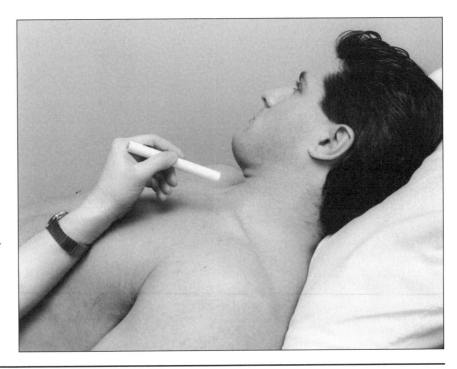

With the patient in the same position, estimate central venous pressure. Begin by palpating the clavicles where they join the sternum (the suprasternal notch). Place your fingers here and slide them down the sternum until you feel a bony protuberance, known as the angle of Louis (or the sternal angle). Place a centimeter ruler vertically (perpendicular to the chest) at this angle. From the ruler, extend a sturdy square-cornered piece of paper horizontally along the highest level of venous pulsation (as shown). Normally, venous pressure is seen below the angle of Louis or less than 4 cm above it.

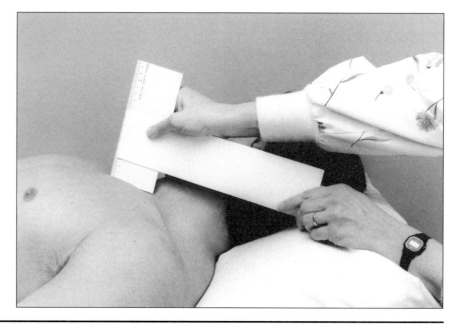

Inspecting the precordium

Have the patient sit on the examination table or stand with his chest exposed so you can inspect his chest and identify the necessary anatomic landmarks.

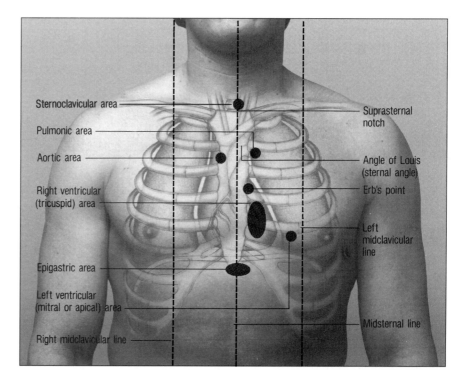

Sternoclavicular area

Pulmonic area

Aortic area

Right ventricular (tricuspid) area

Epigastric area

Left ventricular (mitral or apical) area

Right midclavicular line

Suprasternal notch

Angle of Louis (sternal angle)

Erb's point

Left midclavicular line

Midsternal line

To see lateral landmarks, have the patient raise his arms over his head.

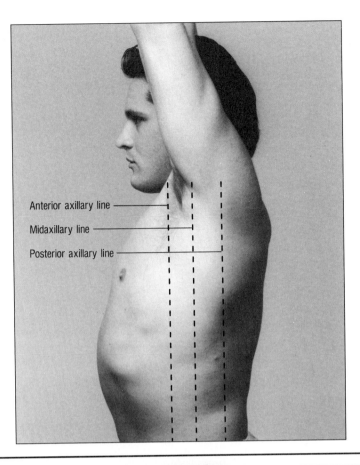

Anterior axillary line

Midaxillary line

Posterior axillary line

Help the patient into the supine position. If he can't tolerate this position, raise his head slightly. Standing by his side—usually his right side—mentally note the anatomic landmarks. Then position the light source (your penlight or gooseneck lamp, for example) so that it again provides indirect light. You should see shadows across the patient's chest. These will help you detect cardiac pulsations.

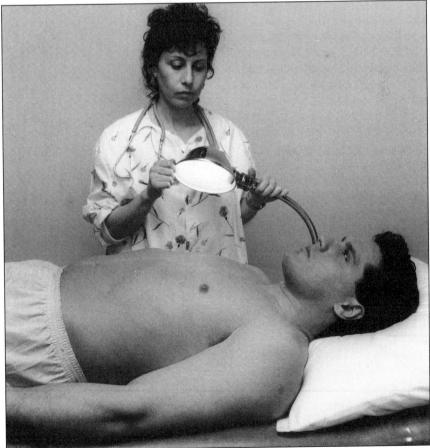

Observe the patient's chest for the apical impulse (pulsations at the apex of the heart). This normally appears in the fifth intercostal space at, or just medial to, the left midclavicular line (left ventricular area). This impulse reflects the location and size of the left ventricle. It usually occupies only one intercostal space.

▷ *Clinical tip:* If a female patient has large breasts, displace them so that you can see the apical impulse. If a patient's chest is enlarged from obesity or emphysema, have him sit up. This position enhances pulsations.

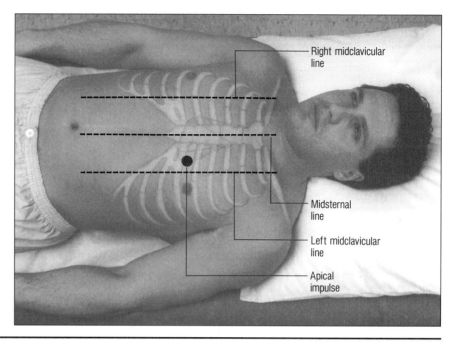

Right midclavicular line

Midsternal line

Left midclavicular line

Apical impulse

Palpating the precordium

Palpate the apical impulse in the left ventricular area. Place your fingertips or the ball of your hand (the palmar surface at the base of the fingers) at the fifth intercostal space, left midclavicular line. This is called the point of maximum impulse (PMI). Light palpation should reveal a tap with each heartbeat. If palpation discloses a weak, an unusually forceful, or a displaced apical impulse, notify the doctor. These are abnormal findings.

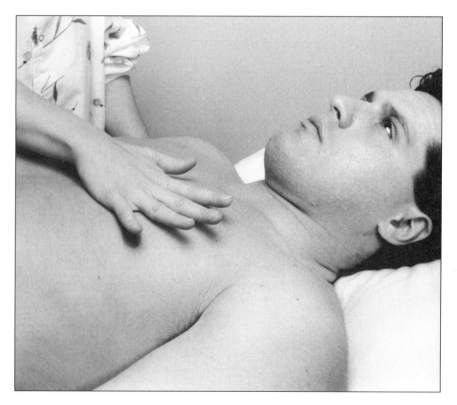

Systematically palpate the sterno-clavicular, aortic, pulmonic, and right ventricular areas for pulsations. Normally, pulsations aren't palpable in these areas. However, in some patients, palpation reveals a vibration that feels like a cat purring. These sensations are heart murmurs (or thrills).

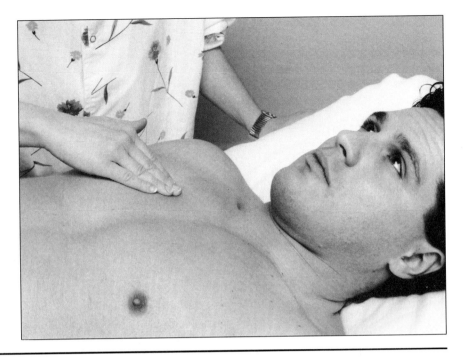

Percussing the precordium

To judge heart size, percuss the heart's borders. Begin at the anterior left axillary line, and percuss toward the sternum in the fifth intercostal space. Note the changes from resonance to dullness (usually near the PMI). If the border extends to the midclavicular line, the left ventricle may be enlarged. On the chest's right side, the heart lies under the sternum and can't be percussed.

▶ *Clinical tip:* If possible, refer to the patient's chest X-ray, which reliably reveals heart size.

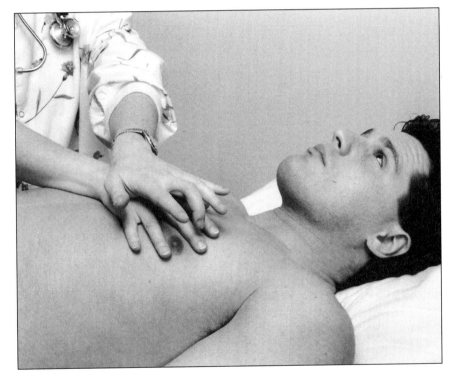

Auscultating the heart

Keep the patient covered and supine, with his head level or slightly elevated. Expose the area to be auscultated. Then warm your stethoscope between your hands (as shown). Have the patient inhale normally through his nose and exhale by mouth.

▶ *Clinical tip:* Don't auscultate through clothing or dressings, which block sound. Also avoid extra noise by keeping the stethoscope tubing off the patient's body or other surfaces.

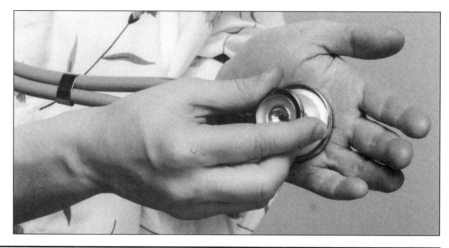

To measure the apical pulse rate, place the diaphragm of the stethoscope over the PMI. Then count the heartbeats for 1 minute.

▶ *Clinical tip:* Note the heart rhythm during this time. Is it regular or irregular? If it's irregular, does the rhythm have a pattern? If so, note the pattern.

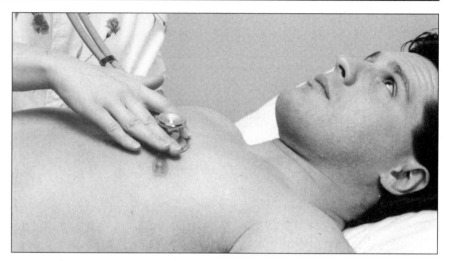

Auscultating normal heart sounds

Mentally identify the four cardiac auscultation sites (shown here in the upright, frontal view to aid visualization). Listen at each site in this sequence: aortic area (second intercostal space, right sternal border), pulmonic area (second intercostal space, left sternal border), mitral area (fifth intercostal space, midclavicular line), and tricuspid area (fifth intercostal space, left sternal border). Because the opening and closing of the heart valves create most normal heart sounds, auscultation sites lie close together in the chest, behind or to the left of the sternum. Auscultation sites are not located directly over the valves; they lie over the pathways the blood takes as it flows through them.

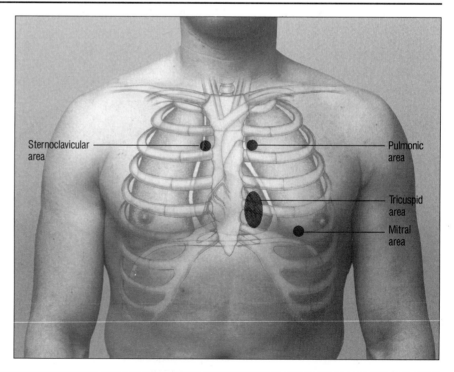

With the patient still supine, place the diaphragm of the stethoscope on one of the auscultation sites. Listen to several cardiac cycles to become familiar with the rate and rhythm of S_1 and S_2. Normal heart sounds last a fraction of a second and are followed by slightly longer silences. Listen closely to these sounds. Their timing in the cardiac cycle tells you how well each valve works.

▶ *Clinical tip:* Always identify S_1 and S_2 first because you need to be familiar with normal sounds before you can identify abnormal ones.

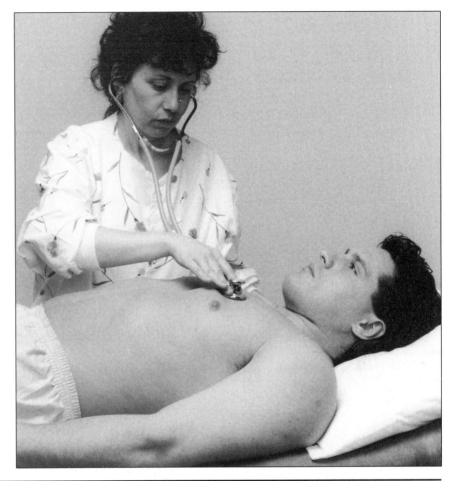

Once you're familiar with the rate and rhythm of normal heart sounds, listen for the heart sounds in each of the four areas following the sequence described previously. First, pressing firmly, use the diaphragm of the stethoscope (as shown). Then, pressing lightly, use the bell.

Note: In the aortic area (shown) and the pulmonic area, S_1 is normally quieter than S_2. A split S_2 may be heard during inspiration in the pulmonic area. In the tricuspid and mitral areas, S_1 is normally louder than S_2. A split S_2 may be heard in the tricuspid area.

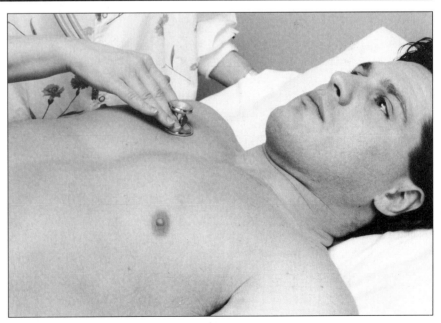

If you have difficulty distinguishing S_1 from S_2, try palpating the carotid artery as you auscultate. S_1 occurs almost simultaneously with the beat of the carotid pulse.

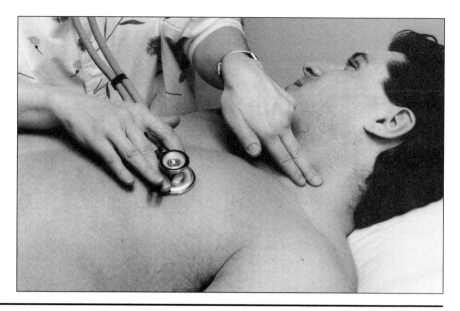

Alternatively or additionally, you can listen to heart sounds with the patient in a left lateral recumbent position. Although S_1 and S_2 are clearly heard with the patient in this position, you'll find this position best for auscultating low-pitched sounds associated with atrioventricular problems, such as mitral valve murmurs and extra heart sounds. To detect these sounds, place the bell over the apical area.

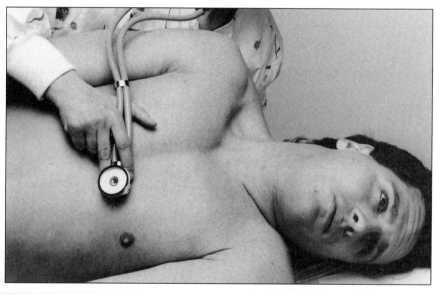

Another alternative or additional way to hear heart sounds is to place the patient in the forward-leaning position. With the patient in this position, you can clearly hear not only normal sounds but also high-pitched sounds related to semilunar valve problems, such as aortic and pulmonic valve murmurs.

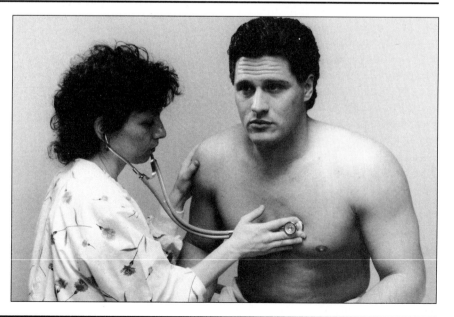

Auscultating additional heart sounds

When auscultating for S_1 and S_2, you may hear additional heart sounds: S_3, S_4, or both. Listen for S_3 (also called a ventricular gallop) when the patient is in the left lateral recumbent position. Place the bell of the stethoscope at the tricuspid and mitral areas. Expect to hear S_3 during early to mid-diastole, just after S_2, at the end of ventricular filling. If the right ventricle is noncompliant, you'll hear the sound in the tricuspid area; if the left ventricle is noncompliant, you'll hear the sound in the mitral area.

▶ *Clinical tip:* The rhythm of S_3 resembles a horse galloping; its cadence resembles the word *ken-tuc-ky* or *lub-dub-by.*

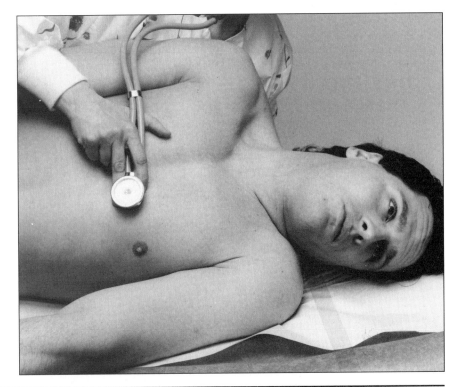

Listen for S_4 (also called atrial or presystolic gallop) with the patient in the supine position. Place the bell of the stethoscope on the patient's chest over the tricuspid and mitral areas. Expect to hear this heart sound late in diastole, immediately before the S_1 of the next cycle. S_4 is associated with the acceleration and deceleration of blood entering a chamber that resists additional filling. In right ventricular dysfunction, you'll hear S_4 in the tricuspid area; in left ventricular dysfunction, you'll hear it in the mitral area.

▶ *Clinical tip:* S_4 has the same cadence as the word *tennes-see* or *le-lub-dub.*

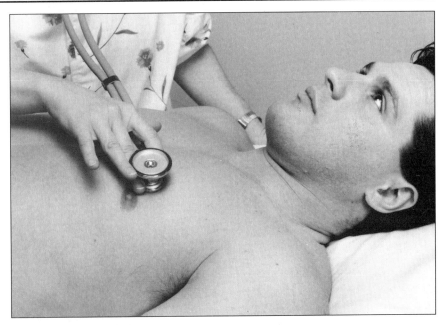

To detect a pericardial friction rub, have the patient sit upright and lean forward or exhale. This enhances the sound of the friction rub. Then use the diaphragm of the stethoscope to auscultate at the third left intercostal space along the lower left sternal border. Listen for a harsh, scratchy, scraping or squeaking sound.

▶ **Clinical tip:** If possible, have the patient hold his breath for a few seconds while you listen. This can eliminate noisy respiratory sounds that may interfere with auscultating for rubs. A rub usually indicates pericarditis.

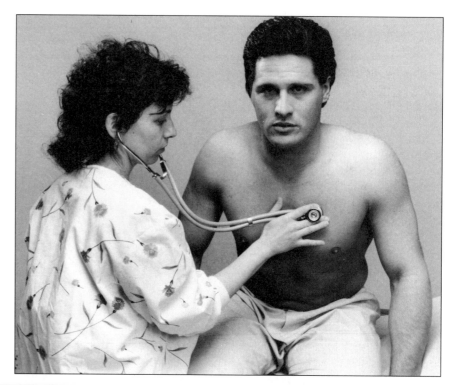

To detect a carotid artery bruit, auscultate each carotid artery by lightly placing the bell of the stethoscope over the carotid artery—first on one side of the trachea, then on the other side. Normally, you should hear no vascular sounds. If you detect a blowing, swishing sound, this usually indicates turbulent blood flow, which may occur in persons who have cardiovascular disease.

▶ **Clinical tip:** Ask the patient to hold his breath, if he can. This will eliminate respiratory sounds that may interfere with your findings.

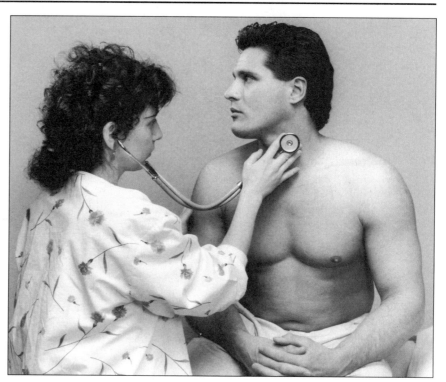

Understanding normal heart sounds in the cardiac cycle

The cardiac cycle has two phases: systole, when the ventricles contract, increasing blood pressure and ejecting blood into the aorta and the pulmonary artery; and diastole, when the ventricles relax and blood pressure decreases, thereby contracting the atria. Using your stethoscope, you can hear each phase reverberate distinctively as the heart's valves open and close.

Sounds of systole

At the beginning of systole, increasing ventricular pressure forces the mitral and tricuspid valves to shut. The closing of these atrioventricular (AV) valves produces the first heart sound (S_1), or the *lub* of *lub-dub.* The ventricular pressure builds until it exceeds that in the pulmonary artery and the aorta. Then the aortic and pulmonic (semilunar) valves open and the ventricles eject blood into the arteries (see arrows below).

Sounds of diastole

As the ventricles empty and relax, ventricular pressure falls below that in the pulmonary artery and the aorta. The semilunar valves close, producing the second heart sound (S_2), or the *dub* of *lub-dub,* and marking the end of systole. As the ventricles relax during diastole, the pressure in the ventricles is less than that in the atria. The AV valves open, and blood begins to flow into the ventricles from the atria (see arrows below). When the ventricles become full near the end of diastole, the atria contract to send the rest of the blood to the ventricles. Ventricular pressure is now greater than atrial pressure. The AV valves close, marking the beginning of systole and repetition of the cardiac cycle.

Note: Events on the right side of the heart occur a fraction of a second after events on the left side because the pressure is lower on the right side of the heart.

Systole

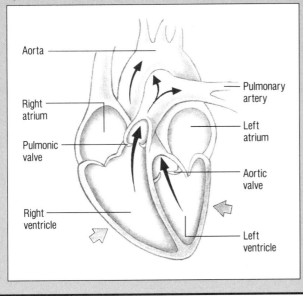

Diastole

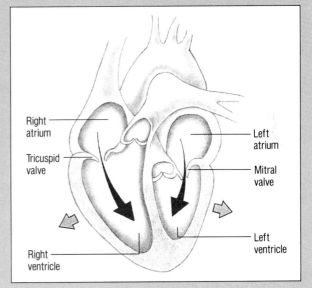

Recognizing abnormal heart sounds

Whenever auscultation reveals an abnormal heart sound, you'll need to identify the sound and its timing in the cardiac cycle. Knowing these characteristics helps you identify the possible cause as described in the chart below.

ABNORMAL HEART SOUND	CYCLICAL TIMING	POSSIBLE CAUSES
Accentuated S_1	Beginning of systole	Mitral stenosis; fever
Diminished S_1	Beginning of systole	Mitral regurgitation; severe mitral regurgitation with calcified, immobile valve; heart block
Split S_1	Beginning of systole	Right bundle-branch block
Accentuated S_2	End of systole	Pulmonary or systemic hypertension
Diminished or inaudible S_2	End of systole	Aortic or pulmonic stenosis
Persistent S_2 split	End of systole	Delayed closure of the pulmonic valve, usually from overfilling of the right ventricle, causing prolonged systolic ejection time
Reversed or paradoxical S_2 split that appears in expiration and disappears in inspiration	End of systole	Delayed ventricular stimulation; left bundle-branch block or prolonged left ventricular ejection time
S_3 (ventricular gallop)	Early diastole	Overdistention of ventricles in rapid-filling segment of diastole; mitral insufficiency or ventricular failure (normal in children and young adults)
S_4 (atrial or presystolic gallop)	Late diastole	Forceful atrial contraction from resistance to ventricular filling late in diastole (resulting from left ventricular hypertrophy), pulmonic stenosis, hypertension, coronary artery disease, or aortic stenosis
Pericardial friction rub (grating or leathery sound at left sternal border; usually muffled, high-pitched, and transient)	Throughout systole and diastole	Pericardial inflammation

EXAMINING THE BREASTS

Whether your patient is male or female, a breast evaluation should be an integral part of your physical assessment. To assess the breasts effectively, compile a careful health history and perform a thorough physical examination. Be sure to explore any breast cancer risk factors, such as a family history of the disease. (See *Exploring breast complaints and cancer risks.*)

As you proceed, keep basic breast anatomy and function in mind. Recognize that breast size and composition vary among individuals according to their age, sex, heredity, and other factors. For example, endocrine changes during pregnancy or

throughout the menstrual cycle can affect breast size and composition. (See *Anatomy of the breasts,* page 94.)

Be sure to emphasize the patient's own role in breast health, especially in detecting changes that suggest possible disease. Show the patient how to perform a breast self-examination. Then, if possible, have the patient repeat the demonstration so that you can correct any errors, encourage compliance, and reinforce your teaching.

ASSESSMENT CHECKLIST

Exploring breast complaints and cancer risks

To help detect breast cancer early, carefully note your patient's health history and complaints. A leading killer of women ages 35 to 54, breast cancer occurs in about 1 in 9 women. About 70% of cases develop in women over age 50. Men may also develop breast cancer, but women are at greatest risk.

Besides age, heredity, and a history of breast cancer, the following factors may place women at increased risk: long menstrual cycle, early onset of menses, late menopause, first pregnancy after age 35, high-fat diet, endometrial or ovarian cancer, radiation exposure, antihypertensive therapy, and alcohol and tobacco use. Keeping these risk factors in mind, ask questions similar to those that follow.

Menstrual history
☐ At what age did you begin menstruating?
☐ Does your period come at regular intervals? How often do you get your period?
☐ How many days does your period usually last? Is your menstrual flow heavy or light? Do you have any breast symptoms before or during menstruation, such as pain, discomfort, tenderness, or nipple discharge?
☐ Have you gone through menopause? If so, when?

Pregnancy history
☐ Have you ever been pregnant? If so, how old were you at each pregnancy?

☐ What was the delivery or termination date for each pregnancy?

Related health history
☐ Have you seen or felt any changes in your breasts? If so, can you describe them?
☐ Do you ever have breast tenderness, tingling, pain, or discharge? Do these symptoms occur regularly or within any pattern? Where and when do they occur?
☐ Have you ever had breast aspiration or biopsy? If so, when and for what reason?
☐ Have you ever had breast surgery, including cosmetic procedures, such as implants, reduction, or augmentation? If so, when and why?
☐ Have you ever been diagnosed with such conditions as breast cancer, fibroadenoma, or fibrocystic breasts?
☐ Have you ever used or are you using any hormonal medications, such as estrogen or progesterone? If so, can you name the medication? How long did you use it? Do you remember your dosage? Are you still taking it? Why did the doctor prescribe it?
☐ Have you ever had a mammogram? If so, when? What were the results?
☐ Did your mother, maternal grandmother, maternal aunt, daughter, or sisters ever have breast cancer? If so, was it in one breast or both? Did it occur before or after menopause?
☐ Do you perform a monthly breast self-examination?

Eileen Suida, RN, and *Kathleen Palilonis, RN,* contributed to this section. Ms. Suida is a perinatal nurse with Healthdyne Perinatal Services, Horsham, Pa. Ms. Palilonis is a staff nurse in the Ob-Gyn Center at Abington (Pa.) Memorial Hospital. The publisher thanks *M.S. Kodsi, MD,* of Abington (Pa.) Memorial Hospital and *Hill-Rom,* Batesville, Ind., for their help.

Anatomy of the breasts

As you examine the breasts, try to visualize the structures that you'll palpate. The breasts lie vertically between the second or third and the sixth or seventh ribs on the anterior chest wall over the pectoralis major and the serratus anterior muscles and horizontally between the sternal border and the midaxillary line.

Breast composition

In women, the breast is a modified sebaceous gland with a centrally located nipple of pigmented erectile tissue ringed by an areola that's darker than the adjacent tissue. Sebaceous glands (Montgomery's tubercles) are scattered on the areolar surface, with hair follicles appearing peripherally.

Beneath the skin are glandular, fibrous, and fatty (adipose) tissues in proportions that vary by age, weight, and other factors such as pregnancy.

A small triangle of tissue, called the tail of Spence, projects into the axilla. Around each breast are 12 to 25 glandular lobes containing acini (or alveoli), which produce milk. These cells empty into the lactiferous ducts that transport milk to the nipple.

Attached to the chest wall musculature are fibrous bands (Cooper's ligaments) that support each breast. Fat makes up the rest of the breast and lies primarily behind and above the glandular lobes.

In men, the breast has a nipple, an areola, and mostly flat tissue contiguous with the adjacent chest.

The lymph nodes

The breast holds several lymph node chains, each of which serves a different area. The pectoral (anterior) lymph nodes drain most of the breast and anterior chest wall.

The brachial (lateral) nodes drain most of the arm. The subscapular (posterior) nodes drain part of the arm and the posterior chest wall. The midaxillary (central) nodes lie near the ribs and serratus anterior muscle, high in the axilla. The pectoral, brachial, and subscapular nodes drain into the midaxillary nodes.

In women, internal mammary nodes, too deep to palpate, drain the mammary lobules, whereas the superficial lymphatic vessels drain the skin. Breast cancer typically spreads via the lymphatic system.

Lateral cross section of female breast

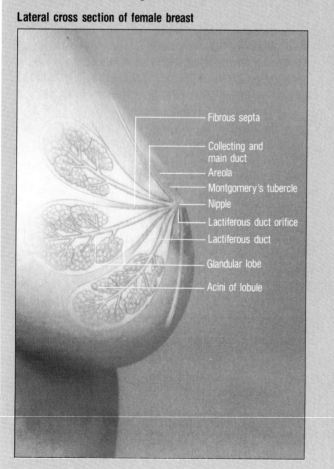

Fibrous septa
Collecting and main duct
Areola
Montgomery's tubercle
Nipple
Lactiferous duct orifice
Lactiferous duct
Glandular lobe
Acini of lobule

Lymph nodes

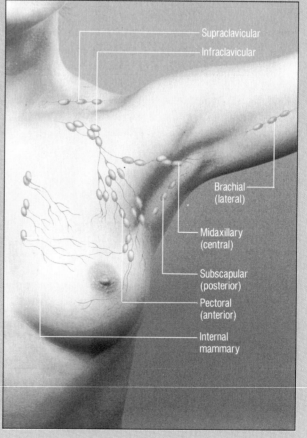

Supraclavicular
Infraclavicular
Brachial (lateral)
Midaxillary (central)
Subscapular (posterior)
Pectoral (anterior)
Internal mammary

Inspecting the breasts

Before beginning, gather the equipment needed for a thorough assessment: a small pillow or a folded towel, a glass slide, and cytologic fixative spray. Nonsterile gloves are optional. You may also need a light source and a ruler calibrated in centimeters.

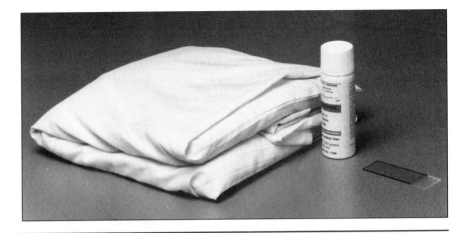

Ask the patient to disrobe to the waist and to sit with her arms resting at each side. First, inspect the breasts for size and symmetry.

▶ *Clinical tip:* In women, the breasts are normally symmetrical, convex, and similiar in appearance. However, one breast (usually the left) may be slightly larger than the other. The male breast may be convex if the patient is overweight or if he's an adolescent with gynecomastia (which typically resolves in about 1 year).

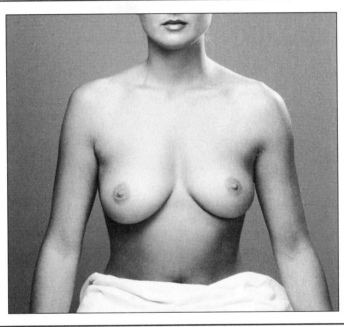

Examine the breasts for obvious masses, one-sided flattening, or retraction or dimpling (a localized depression). To inspect for hidden dimpling, ask the patient to place her hands on her hips (as shown).

Evaluate the skin, which should appear smooth and soft with a similar venous pattern in both breasts. (Pronounced bilateral venous patterns are normal in obese or fair-skinned people.) If you see a skin lesion, ask about its duration and any recent changes. Don't be concerned about unchanged, nontender, and long-standing surface lesions such as nevi.

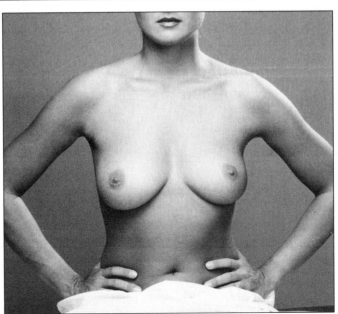

Ask the patient to raise her hands slowly over her head. Inspect for equal and free breast movement without dimpling. Repeat this part of the examination if you are unsure of your findings.

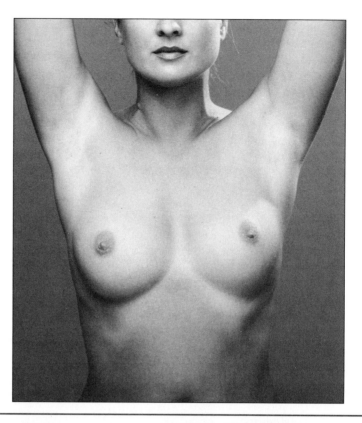

Ask the patient with large or pendulous breasts to stand and lean forward with her hands or arms outstretched (as shown). Support her arms or have her lean on a chair or a table. Both breasts should swing forward freely. This position helps reveal breast or nipple asymmetry that wasn't visible before.

Clinical tip: In pregnant patients, large or pendulous breasts are normal. Other normal inspection findings include enlarged, erectile nipples (flattening or inverting as pregnancy progresses); colostrum secretion; dark, broadened areolae; prominent Montgomery's tubercles; vascular bluish chest veins (from increased estrogen production); and striae from stretching.

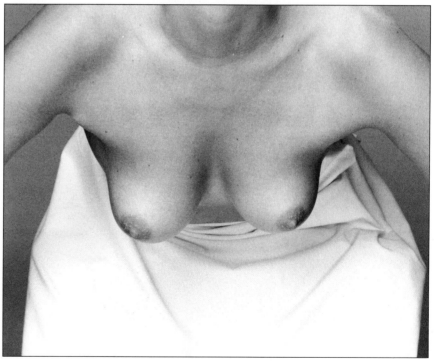

Inspect the nipples and areolae. Assess their size, shape, and color. (In a lactating patient, assess for signs of mastitis.) Normally, the nipples and areolae are similarly round or oval, of equal size, and free of rashes, fissures, or ulcerations. The nipples usually point in the same direction: outward, slightly upward, or laterally.

▶ *Clinical tip:* Inspect Montgomery's tubercles for discharge. A manually expressed discharge can occur normally; a spontaneous discharge is an abnormal finding.

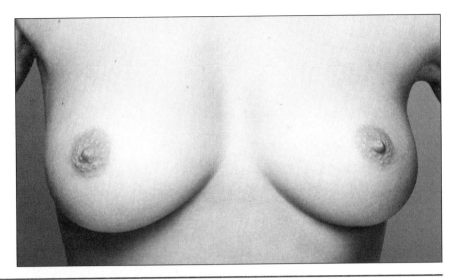

If the patient has had a mastectomy, inspect the scar closely. Malignant changes commonly occur at this site. Look for lumps, color changes, swelling, rash, or irritation. Also assess for muscle loss or lymphedema. If the patient has had breast reconstruction, augmentation, or lumpectomy, inspect the breast in the usual manner. Pay close attention to scar tissue or any other new tissue.

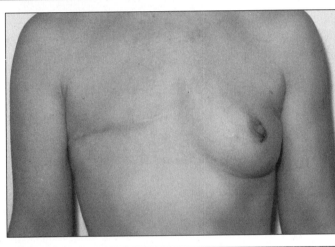

Inspecting and palpating the axillae

While the patient is sitting, inspect the axillae for rashes, signs of infection (such as boils), and unusual pigmentation. Both axillae should be free of rashes or lesions and have hair growth if the patient is past puberty.

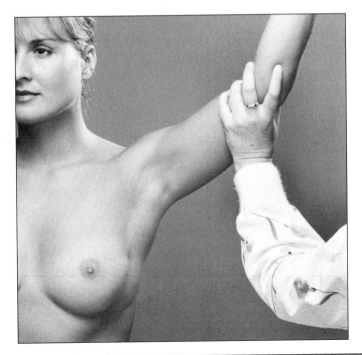

To palpate the axillae, the patient can lie down or sit, but sitting provides easier access. If the patient has an obvious ulceration or nipple discharge, you should wear gloves; otherwise, gloves may interfere with your findings. Ask her to relax her arm as you support her elbow or wrist with one hand.

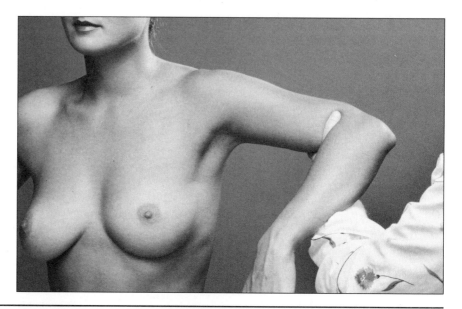

Keeping the fingers of your other hand together, reach high into the apex of the axilla. Position your fingers so that they're directly behind the pectoral muscles, pointing toward the midclavicle. Sweep your fingers downward and against the ribs and the serratus anterior muscle to palpate the midaxillary (central) lymph nodes.

▶ *Clinical tip:* Palpation of one or two small, nontender, freely movable nodes is a normal finding. Hard, large, or tender nodes, however, may be abnormal, as may a suspicious-looking lesion.

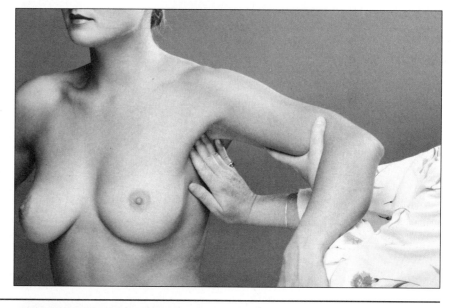

Assess the pectoral (anterior) nodes by palpating along the anterior axillary fold (as shown). Use one hand to provide support under the patient's arm. Use the other hand to grasp the axillary fold between your thumb and fingers, palpating inside the borders of the pectoral muscle.

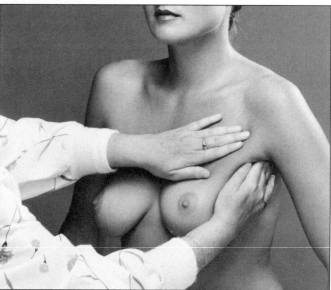

Palpate the brachial (lateral) nodes by pressing your fingers along the upper inner arm, trying to compress these nodes against the humerus.

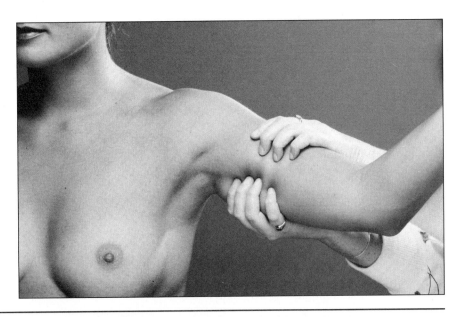

Assess the subscapular (posterior) nodes by palpating along the posterior axillary fold. To do this, stand at the patient's side, and use your fingers to feel inside the muscle of the posterior axillary fold.

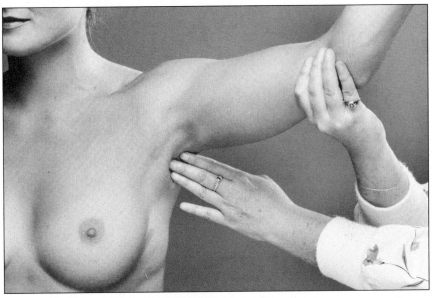

If the axillary node findings appear abnormal, assess the nodes in the clavicular area. Encourage the patient to relax so that her clavicles drop. Direct her to flex her head slightly forward to relax the neck muscles. Then, standing in front of her, hook your fingers over the clavicle beside the sternocleidomastoid muscle. Rotate your fingers deeply into this area to feel the supraclavicular nodes.

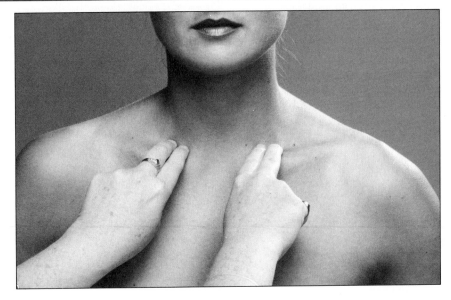

Palpating the breasts

Mentally divide the breasts into four quadrants and a fifth segment, the tail of Spence, so that you can describe your findings according to a quadrant or a segment. Or think of the breast as a clock, with the nipple in the center. Then specify a lesion's location according to the time (2 o'clock, for example). Whether you use the quadrant or clock method, also specify the lesion's location by its distance in centimeters from the nipple.

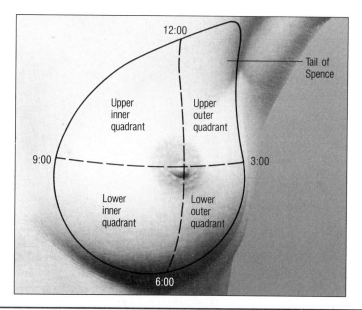

For a supine examination, place a small pillow or folded towel under the patient's back on the side being examined. Then place the arm on that same side above her head. This allows the breast tissue to spread more evenly across the chest wall.

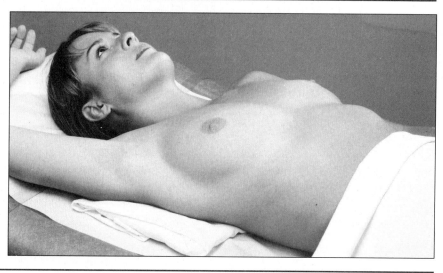

Using your middle three finger pads, which are more sensitive than the fingertips, palpate the breast systematically, rotating your fingers gently against the chest wall (as shown). Palpate each breast circularly from the center out or from the periphery in, making sure to palpate the tail of Spence. Feel for masses or induration (hardness). If you suspect a mass, move or compress the breast gently to look for dimpling. Palpate for consistency and elasticity.

▶ *Clinical tip:* The normal inframammary ridge at the lower edge of the breast is firm and may be mistaken for a tumor.

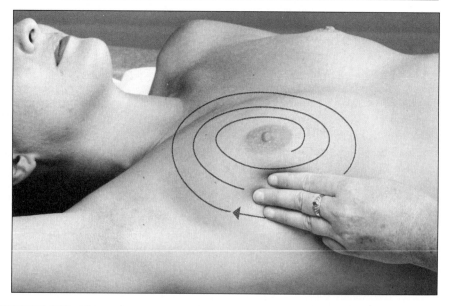

Alternative methods, especially useful in patients with pendulous breasts, are to palpate across or down the breast. For either procedure, ask the patient to sit up. To palpate across the breast, place a supporting hand under the breast while your other hand sweeps down and across the breast tissue against your supporting hand. Repeat this procedure on the other breast.

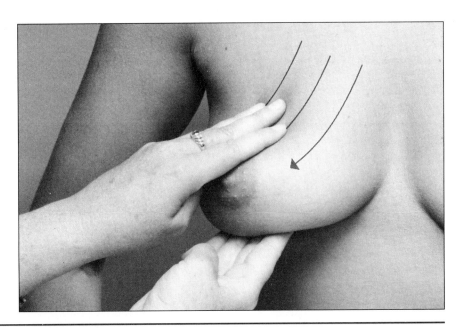

To palpate down the breast, use the finger pads of both hands simultaneously, forming an in-and-out pattern across and down the breast (as shown). Repeat this procedure on the other breast. Also assess for tenderness (which will vary according to the time in the patient's menstrual cycle).

▶ *Clinical tip:* The breasts are typically tender the week before the menstrual period. Note where the patient is in her menstrual cycle when you document breast assessment data.

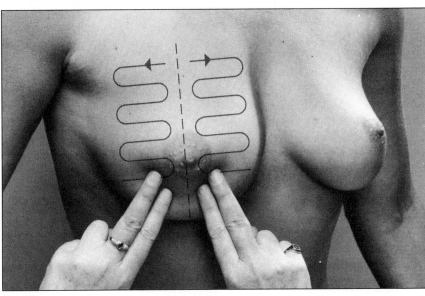

Next, palpate the areolae.

▶ *Clinical tip:* If your patient is male, don't overlook palpation of the areolae and nipples.

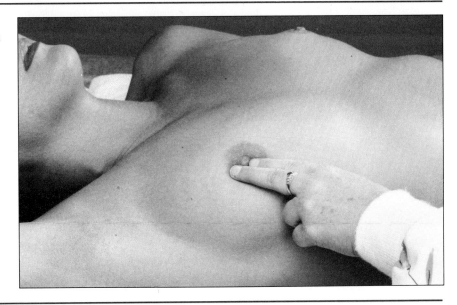

Palpate the nipple by gently compressing it between your thumb and index finger. The nipple will become erect and the areola will pucker from the tactile stimulation. Gently milk the nipple for discharge by compressing it between the thumb and index finger. Repeat this procedure on the other breast. If a discharge occurs, note the duct or ducts through which it appears.

▶ *Clinical tip:* Pregnant or lactating women normally have a discharge during palpation, making milking or squeezing the nipple unnecessary.

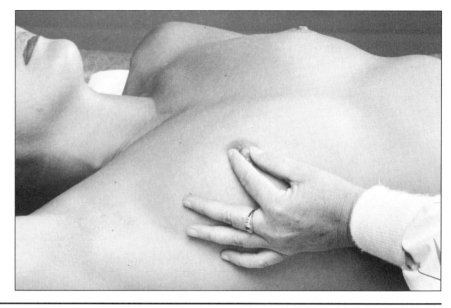

Make a cytologic smear of any discharge not explained by pregnancy or lactation. To do this, put on gloves, and then place a glass slide over the nipple and smear the discharge on the slide.

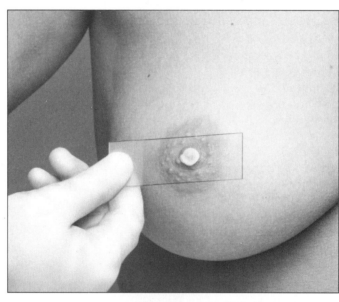

Immediately spray the slide with fixative, making sure to keep the spray nozzle 6″ (15 cm) from the slide. Label the slide with the patient's name and the date, place it in a slide holder and then in a biohazard bag, and send it to the laboratory for analysis.

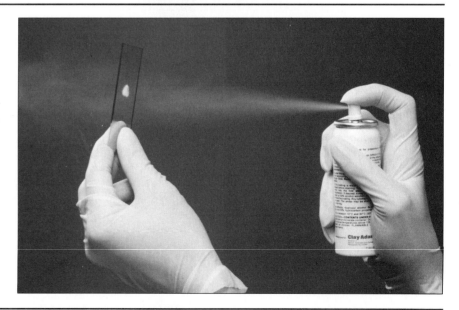

Palpating a breast mass

If you detect a breast mass on palpation, note its size in centimeters, its shape (oval, round, or irregular), and its consistency (for example, firm, cystic, hard, or rubbery).

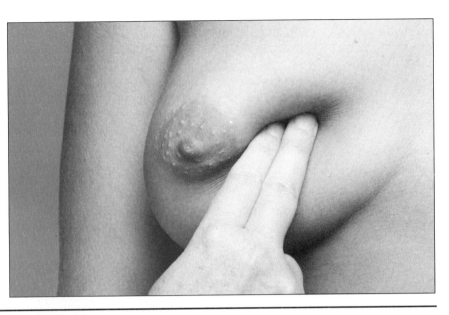

Palpate the mass, delineating it from the surrounding tissue by gently pinching the mass between your thumb and index finger to determine its borders.

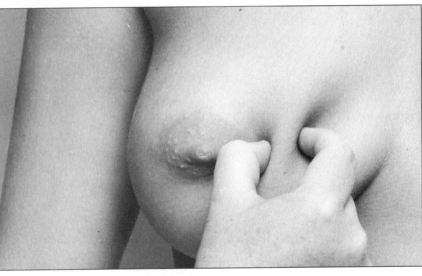

Assess the mass for mobility to determine whether it's fixed to the underlying tissue or freely movable. To do so, gently pinch the mass between your thumb and index finger again, attempting to move the mass back and forth (as shown). Ask the patient if she has any tenderness. Then document the location of the mass by its distance in centimeters from the nipple and its location on the clock (or within the quadrant).

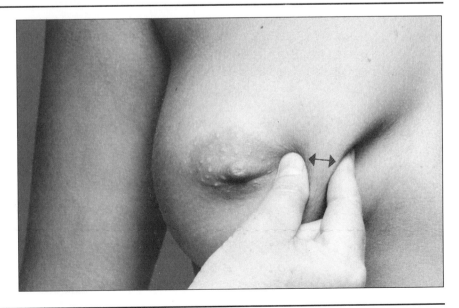

Distinguishing normal from abnormal breast findings

Many breast changes discovered during a routine breast assessment are normal. In young women, breasts will feel firmly elastic with glandular tissue that resembles small lobules. Before menstruation, they may feel unusually nodular and full. In pregnancy, breasts may feel lobular (from hypertrophic mammary alveoli) and during lactation, they'll feel engorged. In mature women, the breasts may feel granular or stringy. With so many normal changes, abnormalities may be difficult to distinguish and interpret. Here are some characteristic abnormal findings.

Breast cysts or masses

In fibrocystic breasts, you may palpate one or more well-defined, movable lumps or cysts. This benign condition results from excess fibrous tissue formation and hyperplasia of the mammary duct linings.

Fibroadenoma, a benign condition, produces a small, round, painless, well-defined, mobile lump that may be soft but is usually solid, firm, and rubbery.

A malignant breast mass usually appears in the upper outer quadrant (although it can occur in any other quadrant) as a hard, immobile, irregular lump. Nipple discharge may occur, and breast skin may become edematous with enlarged pores, discoloration, and an orange-peel appearance (peau d'orange).

Prominent breast veins

Prominent veins may indicate cancer in some patients but may be normal in other patients. Purple striations (which eventually turn silver) may appear also, especially after pregnancy or weight gain.

Breast inflammation

Acute mastitis causes skin abrasions or cracking and reddened skin. Fever and other signs of systemic infection may also occur. The condition is usually associated with lactation. Erythema of the nipple and areola may be an early sign of Paget's disease, a cancer of the mammary ducts. Nipple thickening, scaling, and erosion occur later. Another common sign is a red, scaly, eczema-like rash over the affected nipple and areola.

Nipple retraction and inversion

Retracted (dimpled or creased) areas in the breast skin or nipple result from fibrosis or scar tissue formation and may be a sign of cancer. The breast or nipple may also change contour. You may see retraction upon inspection, or it may not be evident until you palpate or the patient changes position. Inverted nipples may be normal if the patient has always had them. Suspect fibrosis or cancer if inversion occurs suddenly with thickening and broadening of the skin.

Scheduling breast examinations

The American Cancer Society and the American College of Radiology recommend this schedule for regular breast examinations. Depending on their needs, some patients may follow a schedule modified by their doctor.

AGE	BREAST SELF-EXAMINATION	MAMMOGRAPHY	PHYSICAL EXAMINATION
20 to 34	Monthly, 7 to 10 days after menstrual period begins	Not specified	Every 3 years
35 to 39	Monthly, 7 to 10 days after menstrual period begins	One baseline mammogram within this time span	Every 3 years
40 to 49	Monthly, 7 to 10 days after menstrual period begins	Every 1 or 2 years	Yearly
50+	Monthly, 7 to 10 days after menstrual period begins (Postmenopausal women should examine their breasts on the same date each month.)	Yearly	Yearly

EXAMINING THE ABDOMEN

The abdominal cavity houses the liver, spleen, pancreas, gallbladder, stomach, intestines, kidneys, bladder, and other vital structures. It also protects blood vessels, such as the abdominal aorta and the inferior vena cava. Before beginning your physical examination, you should review the location and function of the structures you'll assess (see *Position of abdominal structures,* page 106). Then perform the examination sequence from inspection and auscultation to percussion and palpation over the abdominal quadrants. These include the right upper quadrant (RUQ), the right lower quadrant (RLQ), the left upper quadrant (LUQ), and the left lower quadrant (LLQ). *Note:* Remember to auscultate the abdomen before you percuss and palpate it. Both percussion and palpation commonly affect the normal frequency and vigor of abdominal sounds.

A well-focused health history and a thorough abdominal examination are the chief concerns of any physical assessment—but they're a crucial concern if the patient reports abdominal pain (see *Exploring abdominal complaints,* page 107). Because abdominal pain may signal a life-threatening disorder, you may need to assess your patient quickly.

REVIEWING THE FUNCTION OF G.I. ORGANS

The GI organs normally work together to digest and absorb food and fluids and to eliminate wastes.

The *liver*—the body's largest organ—has a large right lobe and a smaller left lobe, which lie across the abdomen's RUQ and LUQ, respectively. This organ metabolizes carbohydrates, detoxifies harmful substances in plasma, breaks down plasma proteins and amino acids, converts ammonia to urea, and stores iron and vitamins D, K, and B_{12}. It also secretes bile and bilirubin to aid digestion.

Lying horizontally in the RUQ and LUQ behind the stomach, the *pancreas* produces and releases insulin and glycogen, which regulate glucose levels. It also excretes digestive enzymes.

The soft, oval *spleen* lies in the LUQ beneath the diaphragm and behind the lower ribs. This organ destroys old erythrocytes, produces antibodies, and rids the blood of microorganisms.

The *gallbladder,* a small, pear-shaped organ, lies beneath the liver in the RUQ and stores bile until it's needed for digestion.

Located in the LUQ, the J-shaped *stomach* secretes the gastric juices, hydrochloric acid, and enzymes that break down food. It also absorbs small amounts of water, glucose, medication, and alcohol.

The *small intestine*—consisting of the duodenum, the jejunum, and the ileum—lies mainly in the RUQ and the RLQ, although some extends to the LLQ. The small intestine absorbs and digests carbohydrates, fats, and proteins.

Traversing all four quadrants, the *large intestine* consists of the cecum, the appendix, the colon (including the ascending, transverse, descending, and sigmoid portions), the rectum, and the anus. It absorbs nutrients, water, and electrolytes; synthesizes vitamins; and eliminates fecal matter.

REVIEWING THE FUNCTION OF RENAL STRUCTURES

The kidneys, ureters, and bladder constitute the renal system, which purifies the blood and eliminates fluid waste.

The *kidneys* are bean-shaped organs located in the RUQ and the LUQ. The right kidney sits just below the liver; the left kidney sits slightly higher, between the first and fourth lumbar vertebrae. The kidneys regulate fluid and electrolyte balance by glomerular filtration and remove wastes via the urinary tract.

Connecting each kidney to the bladder are foot-long tubules called the *ureters.* Located in each quadrant, the ureters transport urine from the kidneys to the bladder for excretion.

The *bladder,* located medially in both lower quadrants, is an elastic, balloonlike organ that holds urine until it fills to the point of parasympathetic stimulation, resulting in the urge to urinate.

REVIEWING THE FUNCTION OF VASCULAR STRUCTURES

The inferior vena cava and the abdominal aorta are major blood vessels in the abdominal area.

Located in the RLQ and LLQ, the *inferior vena cava* begins at the level of the fourth vertebra and descends into the abdomen. The lumbar, renal, suprarenal, inferior phrenic, and hepatic veins empty into the inferior vena cava.

The *abdominal aorta* branches into the RLQ and LLQ. Beginning at the level of the 12th thoracic vertebra, the abdominal aorta descends into the abdomen and divides into the common iliac arteries.

Lynne Patzek Miller, RN,C, BS, and *Teresa Palmer, RN, MSN, CANP,* contributed to this section. Ms. Miller is operating room manager at Doylestown (Pa.) Hospital. Ms. Palmer is a nurse practitioner in adult cardiac surgery at Robert Wood Johnson University Hospital, New Brunswick, N.J. The publisher thanks *Hill-Rom,* Batesville, Ind., for its help.

Position of abdominal structures

Knowing the location of each abdominal structure and understanding its function will help speed your assessment. To begin, identify the position of each structure in the abdominal quadrants. At the center of these quadrants lies the umbilicus.

Typically, you'll examine GI, renal, and vascular structures during your abdominal assessment.

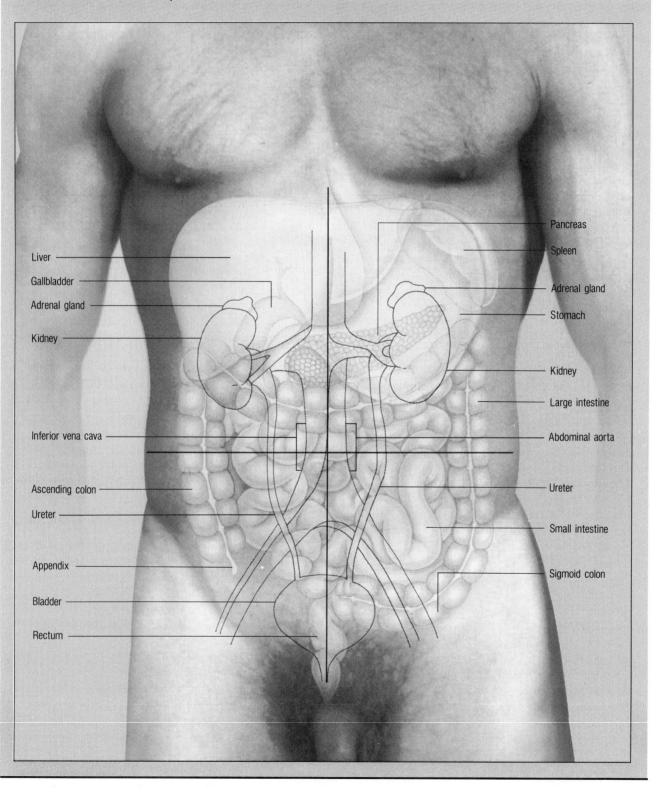

Liver

Gallbladder

Adrenal gland

Kidney

Inferior vena cava

Ascending colon

Ureter

Appendix

Bladder

Rectum

Pancreas

Spleen

Adrenal gland

Stomach

Kidney

Large intestine

Abdominal aorta

Ureter

Small intestine

Sigmoid colon

Exploring abdominal complaints

Before performing an abdominal assessment, take a detailed history. Begin with the patient's chief complaint, which may be related to pain, GI distress, or another problem. Use the following questions as a guide.

Pain history

☐ Do you currently have pain in your abdomen? Can you describe the pain? Is it dull? Throbbing? Fiery?

☐ How often do you have this pain? Does it occur intermittently? Constantly?

☐ What relieves the pain? What worsens it?

GI and related medical history

☐ How is your appetite? Have you noticed a change in it recently?

☐ Have you lost or gained weight recently? If so, how much? Have you been trying to lose weight? Have you ever had a problem either gaining or losing weight?

☐ Do you have indigestion, heartburn, or gas? Does it usually occur after you eat or drink certain foods or beverages? If so, which foods or beverages?

☐ Do you take medication to relieve the discomfort? If so, which medication?

☐ Do you frequently feel nauseated or vomit? What does the vomitus look like? Is it ever dark brown or black?

☐ Have you ever vomited blood?

☐ Do you take any medication for nausea or vomiting? If so, what?

☐ Have you ever been tested or treated for an ulcer? When?

☐ Do you have ulcer pain? Can you describe it?

☐ What triggers or relieves your pain?

☐ How often do you have a bowel movement?

☐ Do you have problems with diarrhea or constipation?

☐ Do you take laxatives or antidiarrheals? If so, which medications? How frequently do you take them?

☐ Do you ever have black stools or blood in your stools? How often? Have you noticed any changes in your bowel habits?

☐ Have you ever had a colon X-ray or a colonoscopic or proctoscopic examination? When? Do you know why you had these tests?

☐ Do you ever have a bladder problem? Can you describe the problem?

☐ Have you ever been tested or treated for a bladder problem? Can you describe the test or treatment?

☐ Do you have hemorrhoids?

☐ When did you last see a doctor for abdominal or intestinal problems?

☐ Have you ever had abdominal surgery? If so, when and what kind?

☐ Do you have a colostomy or an ileostomy? How long have you had it and why was it done?

☐ How do you care for your colostomy or ileostomy?

General medical history

☐ Have you ever been diagnosed with diabetes, stroke, cancer, breathing problems, or bleeding?

☐ What other medical problems do you have?

☐ Are you currently being treated by other doctors? What are their names and specialties? Why are you seeing them?

☐ Are you allergic to any foods or medications?

☐ Are you currently taking any prescription or nonprescription medications? What are their names?

☐ Have you traveled recently? If so, were you outside this country?

Family history

☐ Has anyone in your family been treated for diabetes, stroke, cancer, breathing problems, or any other serious health problem?

☐ Are your grandparents, parents, siblings, or offspring still alive? If so, how is their general health? If not, what did they die of? Has anyone in your family died recently? Of what?

Psychosocial history

☐ What is your occupation?

☐ How would you describe your family life?

☐ How would you describe your stress level?

☐ Do you exercise regularly? What kinds of exercise do you do?

☐ Do you sleep well? How many hours of sleep do you usually need? How many do you get?

Evaluating the abdomen

To begin your assessment, you'll need a sphygmomanometer, a pen or a marker, a cloth tape measure, a centimeter ruler, a safety pin, and a stethoscope. If the patient has abdominal pain, assess the painful area last so that the patient's resultant discomfort doesn't alter the rest of your findings.

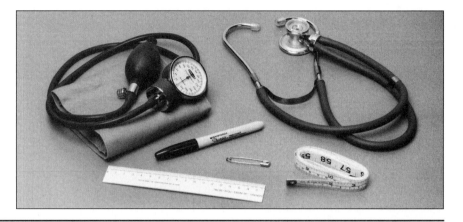

Have the patient void before you begin the examination. Help him into a supine position; then take his vital signs. Explain each procedure before you perform it.

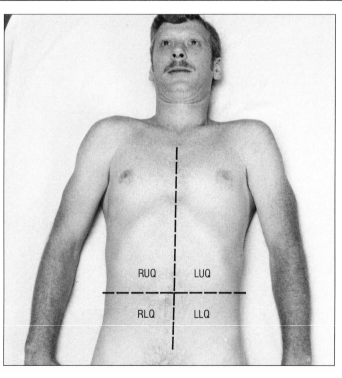

Inspecting the abdomen

Expose the patient's abdomen, and mentally divide it into four quadrants. Observe abdominal shape and symmetry. Inspect the skin for color, striae, rashes, scars, lesions, and hair pattern. Also look for any visible abdominal pulsations. Note the location and contour of the umbilicus.

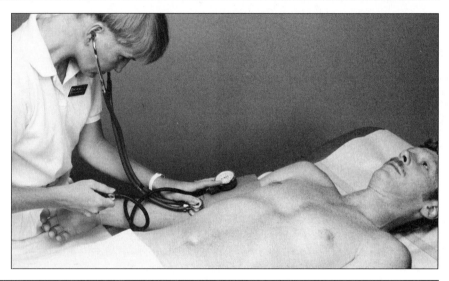

Measure abdominal girth, using a cloth tape measure. A good starting point is the umbilicus. Extend the tape around the patient's back, and return it to the umbilicus. Record this measurement.

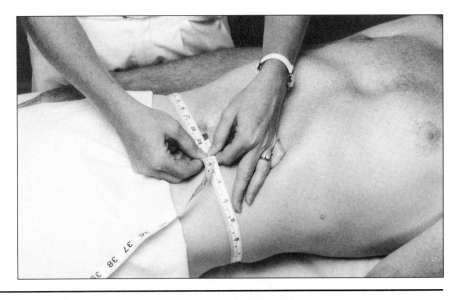

Auscultating the abdomen

Using the diaphragm of the stethoscope, auscultate for bowel sounds. Begin in the RUQ and continue clockwise through the quadrants, listening for at least 2 minutes in each. Note the frequency and intensity of sounds. If you don't hear any sounds after 5 minutes, record bowel sounds as absent.

▶ *Clinical tip:* If the patient has a nasogastric tube connected to suction, turn off the suction before auscultating. Suctioning noises may obscure or replicate actual bowel sounds.

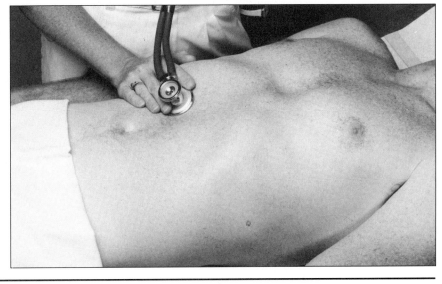

Auscultate for vascular sounds in all four quadrants in the areas shown.

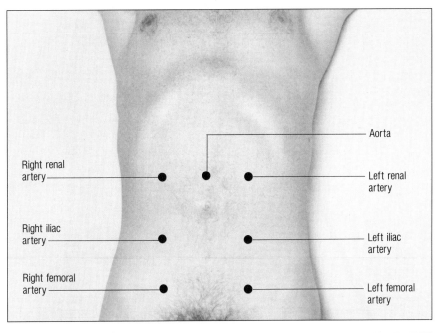

Right renal artery

Aorta

Left renal artery

Right iliac artery

Left iliac artery

Right femoral artery

Left femoral artery

Use the bell of the stethoscope to auscultate for vascular sounds. Listen for hums in the umbilical and epigastric areas and for bruits anywhere in the abdomen.

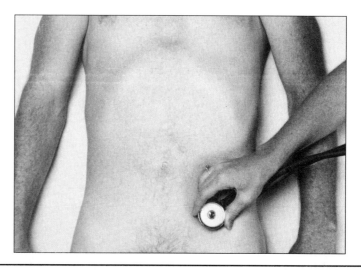

Percussing the abdomen

Use percussion to check the size and location of the patient's abdominal organs. Begin by placing your nondominant hand on the patient's RUQ. Use the tip of the middle finger of your dominant hand to tap the middle finger of your nondominant hand just below the distal point. Move your hands clockwise over the abdomen, mentally picturing the organs in each quadrant.

▶ *Clinical tip:* Don't percuss the abdomen if the patient has an abdominal aortic aneurysm or a transplanted abdominal organ. Doing so may precipitate a rupture.

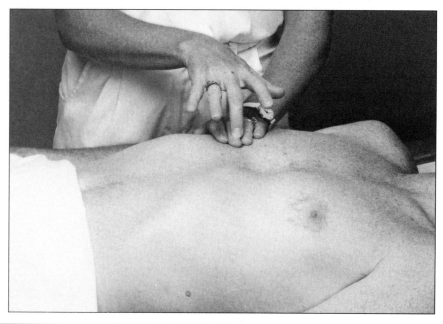

During percussion, be alert for tympanic and dull sensations. Normally, tympany occurs over hollow structures, such as the stomach, intestines, empty bladder, abdominal aorta, and gallbladder. Abnormally high-pitched tympanic sounds suggest bowel distention.

Normally, dull sounds are heard over solid structures, such as the liver, spleen, pancreas, kidneys, and uterus. Be alert for abnormal dullness from solid tumors in the lower abdomen or from ascites.

In a patient with ascites, you're likely to hear tympany in the upper abdomen and dullness in dependent areas.

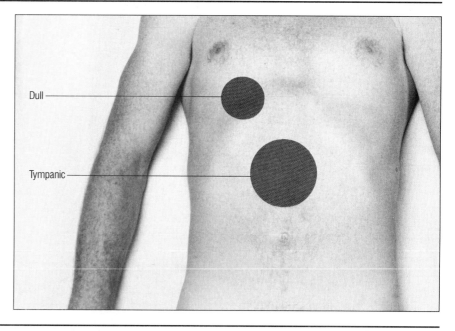

Percuss the liver to help detect an underlying disease such as cirrhosis. Ask the patient to take a deep breath and hold it. Start percussing two fingerbreadths below the right nipple along the midclavicular line. You should sense resonance over the lungs. When resonance changes to dullness, mark the area; this mark indicates the liver's upper border. To find the liver's lower border, start percussing about three fingerbreadths below the umbilicus. Move upward until the sound changes from tympany (over the stomach) to dullness. Mark this spot.

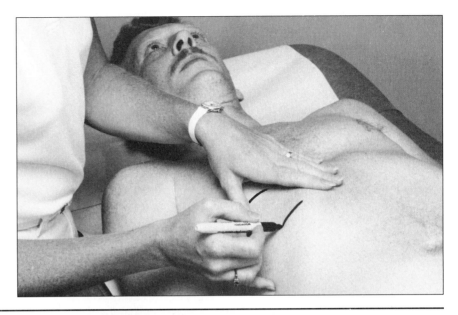

Estimate the size of the liver by measuring the distance between the two marks. A normal span over the liver ranges between 2½" and 5" (6 and 13 cm).

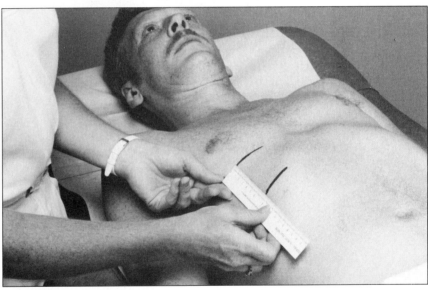

Make sure the patient is properly draped. Percuss the area over the bladder, starting about 2" (5 cm) above the symphysis pubis. Continue percussing downward. A tympanic sound is normal over an empty bladder; a dull sound indicates a distended bladder.

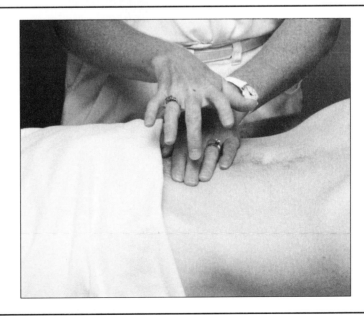

To percuss the spleen, have the patient turn from his back to his right side. Beginning at the sixth rib, percuss posteriorly along the midaxillary line until the sound changes from resonance (from the lungs) to tympany (from colonic or gastric air) over the spleen. Have the patient take deep breaths during the process. Because an enlarged spleen moves forward and downward with inspiration, a descent from tympany to dullness suggests splenic enlargement.

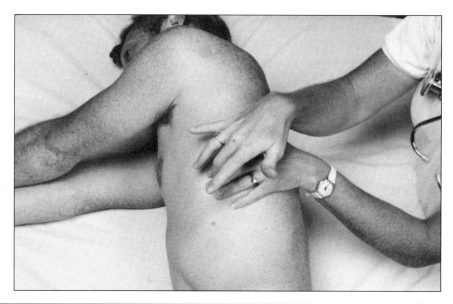

Use blunt percussion to assess for kidney tenderness. Have the patient sit up or lie on his side. Place one hand palm down over the costovertebral angle, between the spine and the 12th rib. Strike this hand lightly with the fist of your other hand. A resonant sound indicates that your hand is over a kidney. If the patient complains of tenderness during this percussion, suspect kidney, liver, or gallbladder inflammation.

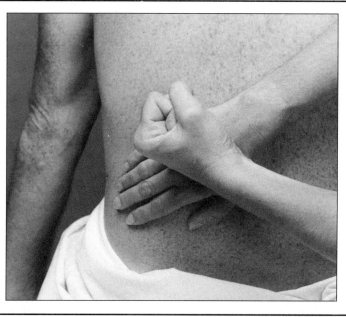

Palpating the abdomen

Use palpation techniques to assess the size, shape, position, and tenderness of major abdominal structures. Ask the patient to keep his abdomen relaxed during the examination. Make sure your hands are warm. Palpate one structure at a time.

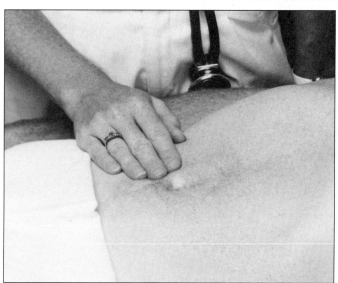

To palpate the liver, slide your left hand under the patient's back, at the approximate location of the liver. Place your right hand below the lower mark that you made to indicate the liver's lower border, and point your fingers toward the right costal margin. Gently press in and up as the patient inhales. The edge of the liver should feel firm, rounded, and smooth. Note any irregularities or tenderness.

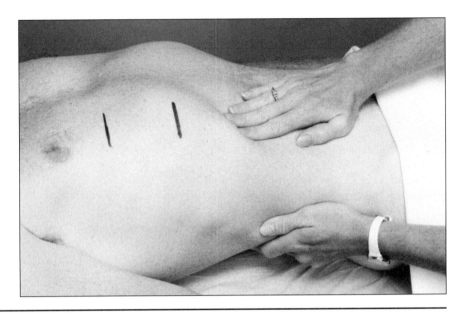

If you can't palpate the liver, try "hooking" it. Stand next to the patient's right shoulder, and place your hands side by side below the lower mark. Ask the patient to take a deep breath. Then press your fingers in and up as you attempt to feel the edge of the liver.

▶ *Clinical tip:* The patient with abdominal pain may be unable to tolerate this procedure.

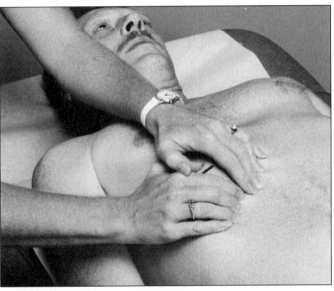

Employing the same palpation technique that you used for the liver, try to palpate the gallbladder (a normal gallbladder isn't palpable). If the gallbladder is enlarged and distended, you'll feel it below the liver margin at the lateral border of the rectus muscle, either medially or laterally. An enlarged, tender gallbladder suggests cholecystitis; an enlarged, nontender gallbladder may signal obstructive disease.

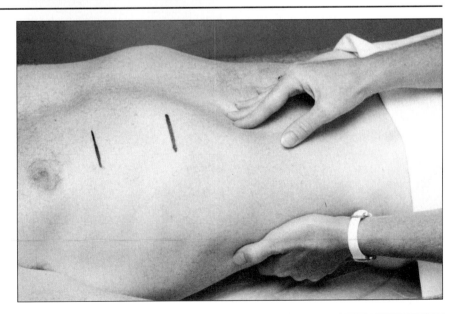

To palpate the spleen, stand on the patient's right side, reach across his abdomen, and use your left hand to support the posterior left lower rib cage. Ask the patient to take a deep breath and hold it while you press up and in toward the left costal margin with your right hand (as shown).

Although a normal spleen isn't palpable, an enlarged spleen is. It's graded by the number of centimeters that it extends below the costal margin. Slight enlargement is 1 to 4 cm; moderate enlargement, between 4 and 8 cm; and great enlargement, more than 8 cm.

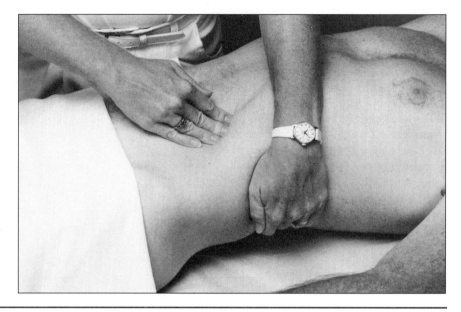

Alternatively, turn the patient on his right side to help bring the spleen down and forward (closer to the abdominal wall), and then palpate similarly (as shown).

▶ **Clinical tip:** If you can't palpate the spleen, don't press too hard—manual compression of an enlarged spleen can rupture it.

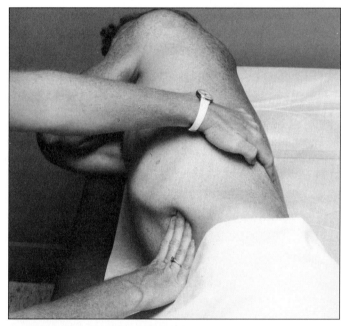

To palpate the right kidney, stand on the patient's right side. Place your left hand under his waist (just below the 12th rib) and your right hand on his abdomen (as shown). Tell him to take a deep breath (so that his kidney will move downward). As he inhales, press up with your left hand and down with your right hand. The kidney should be firm, smooth, and nontender.

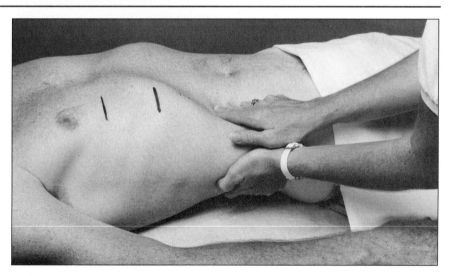

To palpate the left kidney, remain at the patient's right side. Reach across him with your left arm, and place your left hand under his back at waist level. Pull up with your left hand to elevate and displace the kidney anteriorly. Ask the patient to take a deep breath; then try to palpate the lower pole of the left kidney with your right hand. (Note that the left kidney is rarely palpable because it's behind the spleen.)

Alternatively, you may palpate the left kidney from the patient's left side. You'll use the same method described in palpating the right kidney.

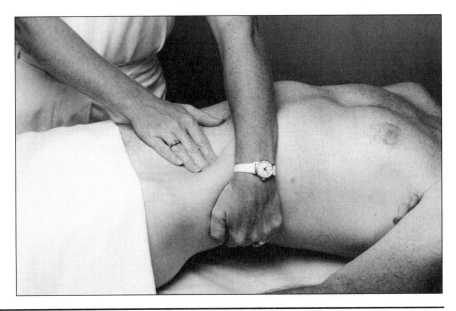

Use bimanual technique to palpate the bladder. Begin at the midline, 1″ to 2″ (2.5 to 5 cm) above the symphysis pubis, and continue palpating until you feel the edge of the bladder. A smooth, rounded, fluctuant suprapubic mass suggests distention; a fluctuant mass extending to the umbilicus indicates extreme distention. A normal bladder may be undetectable.

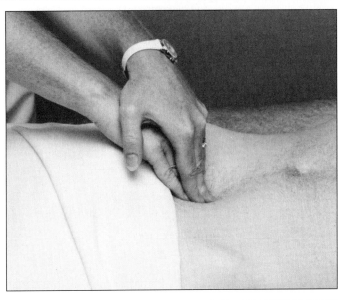

To palpate the abdominal muscles, apply light pressure on the umbilical ring and around the umbilicus. The muscle should feel smooth, with no bulges, nodules, or soft openings (herniations). Continue light palpation of all four quadrants of the abdomen.

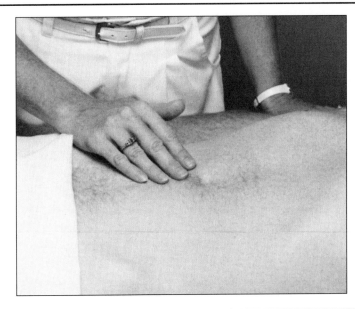

To perform deep palpation of the abdominal muscles, place one hand on top of the other, exerting pressure with the top hand. Observe for tenderness, pulsations, symmetry, mobility, rigidity, guarding, ascites, or pain. Deep palpation may also be used to evaluate abdominal masses. If you detect a mass, note its size, location, shape, and consistency and whether it's tender, fixed, or mobile.

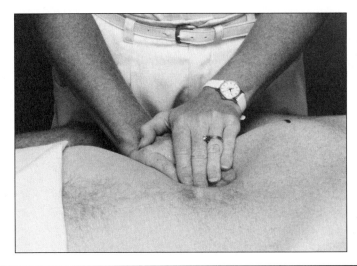

Assessing for additional problems

If you suspect *advanced ascites* (a large accumulation of fluid in the abdominal cavity), have an assistant place her hand and forearm firmly on the patient's abdomen at the midline. Then place the palm of your hand against the patient's left abdomen. Now sharply tap the right abdomen with your fingers. If the patient has advanced ascites, you may see a "fluid wave" ripple across the abdomen.

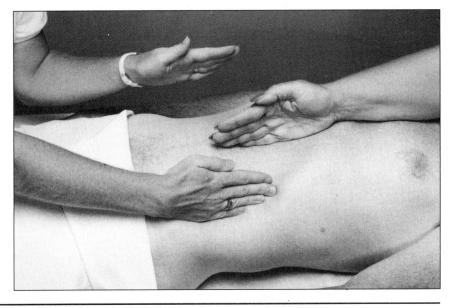

If you suspect *peritoneal irritation,* test for rebound tenderness. With your fingers extended at a 90-degree angle to the abdomen (as shown), press gently and deeply into an area that's not painful. Then rapidly withdraw pressure. The rebound of the compressed structures will cause a sharp, stabbing pain on the side that's irritated. Because this maneuver may increase pain or produce spasms, perform it at the end of your abdominal examination.

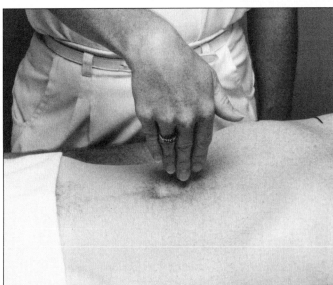

Alternatively, to detect peritoneal irritation, test the subcutaneous sensory nerve fibers for zones of hypersensitivity, which are thought to reflect zones of peritoneal irritation. Lightly stimulate various abdominal areas with a safety pin (near right).

Next, with your thumb and forefinger, gently lift a skinfold away from the abdominal muscle (far right). Repeat this test in various zones. Note the patient's response. (He may grimace or pull away.) Mark the abdominal area where the patient felt discomfort. Document your findings.

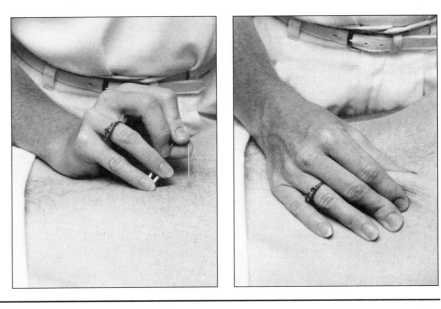

If you suspect that the patient has *appendicitis,* do the iliopsoas muscle test. With the patient in a supine position, place your hand on the anterior surface of his right lower thigh. Then ask the patient to flex his right leg at the hip. As he raises his leg, exert light resistance. Repeat the procedure on the left leg.

If this maneuver causes increased pain in the lower abdominal quadrants, the psoas muscle may be irritated (a sign of an inflamed appendix).

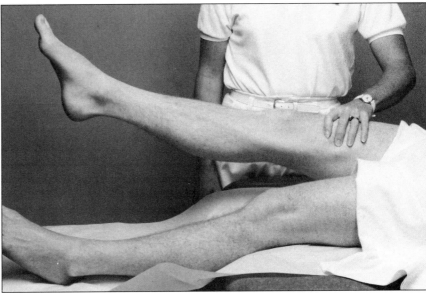

To assess for a *perforated appendix* or a *pelvic abscess,* do the obturator muscle test. Place the patient in a supine position, with his right leg flexed 90 degrees at the knee and hip. Hold the leg just above the knee and ankle, and rotate it laterally and medially. If this maneuver causes increased pain in the hypogastric area, the obturator muscle is irritated, which may signal a perforated appendix or a pelvic abscess.

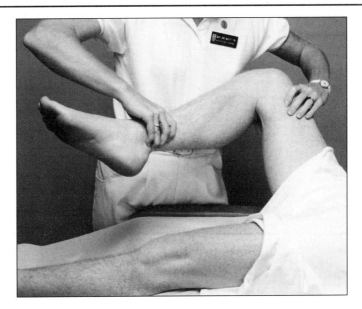

Evaluating abnormal abdominal and bowel sounds

SOUND	LOCATION	POSSIBLE CAUSE
Abdominal sounds		
• Friction rub (harsh grating—like two pieces of sandpaper rubbing together)	• Over liver and spleen	• Inflammation of the liver's peritoneal surface, as occurs from a tumor
• Systolic bruits (vascular blowing sounds that resemble cardiac murmurs)	• Over abdominal aorta	• Partial arterial obstruction or turbulent blood flow
	• Over renal artery	• Renal artery stenosis
	• Over iliac artery	• Hepatomegaly
• Venous hum (continuous, medium-pitched tone of blood flowing in a large, engorged vascular organ such as the liver)	• Epigastric and umbilical regions	• Increased collateral circulation between portal and systemic venous systems, as occurs in hepatic cirrhosis
Bowel sounds		
• Hyperactivity (unrelated to hunger)	• Any quadrant	• Diarrhea or early intestinal obstruction
• Hypoactivity to silence	• Any quadrant	• Paralytic ileus or peritonitis
• High-pitched tinkling	• Any quadrant	• Intestinal fluid and air under tension in a dilated bowel
• High-pitched rushing (coinciding with abdominal cramps)	• Any quadrant	• Intestinal obstruction

EXAMINING THE FEMALE GENITALIA

Assessment of the genitalia requires a thorough understanding of the female reproductive system. (See *Anatomy of the female reproductive system.*) This knowledge forms the basis for obtaining the patient's reproductive health history and carrying out the physical examination. (See *Exploring female reproductive health complaints,* page 121.)

When examining the genitalia, be careful to respect the patient's privacy. Depending on the law in your state, usually only the examiner, possibly the examiner's assistant, and the patient should be in the room. In some cases—for example, with an adolescent—a parent may also stay in the examination room.

Anatomy of the female reproductive system

An accurate physical assessment of the female genitalia depends on understanding external and internal genital structures and function.

External genitalia
Collectively called the vulva, the external genitalia comprises the mons pubis, labia majora, labia minora, clitoris, vaginal introitus, hymen, and Skene's and Bartholin's glands.

The mons pubis is the fatty pad covering the symphysis pubis. After puberty, a patch of coarse, curly hair covers the mons pubis and extends in an inverted triangle to the lower abdomen.

The outer vulvar lips, or labia majora, are two rounded folds of adipose tissue that extend from the mons pubis to the perineum, which is the tissue between the vaginal opening (introitus) and the anus.

The inner vulvar lips are called the labia minora, and their anterolateral and medial parts join to form the prepuce and frenulum of the clitoris. The posterior union of the labia minora is called the fourchette.

The vestibule, the area between the labia minora, contains the clitoris and the vaginal and urethral openings. Composed of sensitive, erectile tissue, the clitoris lies between the labia minora at the top of the

(continued)

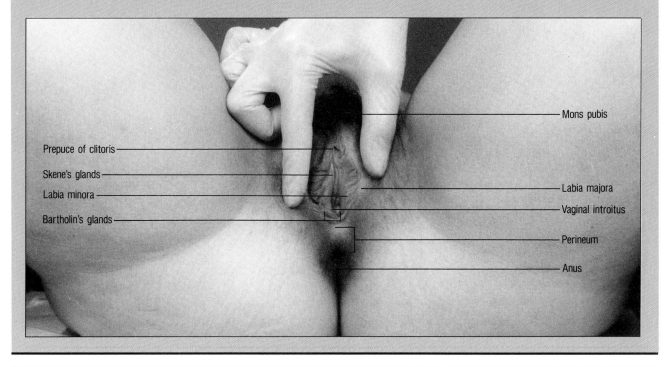

Prepuce of clitoris
Skene's glands
Labia minora
Bartholin's glands
Mons pubis
Labia majora
Vaginal introitus
Perineum
Anus

Teresa Palmer, RN, MSN, CANP, and *Karen E. Michael, RN, MSN,* contributed to this selection. Ms. Palmer is an assistant clinical professor at the University of Medicine and Dentistry of New Jersey in Newark. Ms. Michael is a case manager for Greater Atlantic Health Service, Philadelphia. The publisher thanks *Abington Health Center,* Warminster, Pa., and *Hill-Rom,* Batesville, Ind., for their help.

Anatomy of the female reproductive system *(continued)*

vestibule. The urethral opening (or orifice) is an irregular slit posterior to the clitoris. The vaginal opening is posterior to the urethral orifice. This is a narrow vertical slit in women with intact hymens and a wider opening with irregular edges in women with perforated hymens.

Two kinds of glands have ducts that open into the vulva. Skene's glands are multiple, tiny structures located just below the urethra. Each contains between 6 and 31 ducts. Bartholin's glands lie posterior to the vaginal opening. These glands aren't visible, but both are palpable if they're enlarged.

Internal genitalia

The vagina, cervix, uterus, ovaries, and fallopian tubes make up the internal genitalia. The vagina, a hollow, collapsed tube, extends upward between the urethra and the rectum and back to the uterus. The cup-shaped upper end is the external fornix. About 6″ (15 cm) long in women, the vagina is a highly dilatable passage, facilitating menstruation, sexual intercourse, and childbirth.

The uterus is a hollow, muscular organ divided into the body (the corpus) and the cervix (the narrow, lower end that projects into the vaginal vault). The body's upper convex portion is the fundus; its constricted lower portion is the isthmus, which connects the uterine body to the cervix. The normal position of the uterus is slightly anteflexed, but this position may vary depending on the fullness of the bladder. The only function of the uterus is to house a developing embryo.

The ovaries, a pair of oval-shaped organs about 1¼″ (3 cm) long, are usually found near the lateral pelvic wall at the height of the anterosuperior iliac spine. They produce ova and release the hormones estrogen, progesterone, and testosterone. During puberty, the ovaries stimulate growth of the uterus and its endometrial lining. They also spur vaginal enlargement, epithelial thickening, and secondary sex characteristics.

The two fallopian tubes, each about 4″ (10 cm) long, extend from the ovaries into the upper portion of the uterus. Their funnel-shaped ends curve toward the ovaries, and their fingerlike projections guide the ovum to the uterus after the ovary releases the ovum.

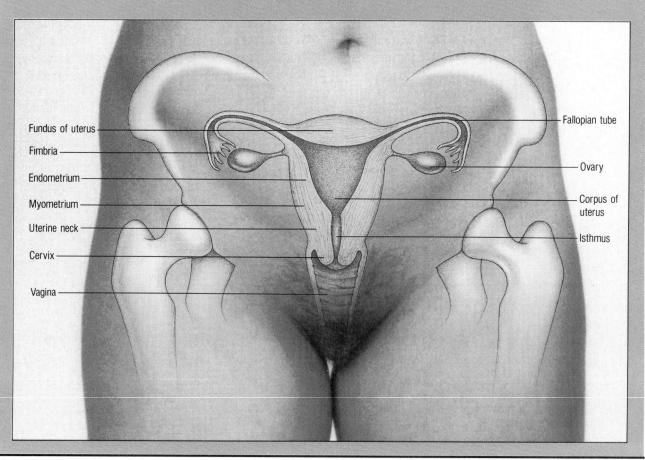

Exploring female reproductive health complaints

To obtain complete reproductive health data, focus first on the patient's current complaints. Then categorize your questions, exploring the patient's reproductive, sexual-social, family, and general health. Use the following questions as a guide.

Current complaint

☐ What brought you in for an examination today? (Guide the patient with more specific questions if she has trouble describing her concerns.)

☐ Can you describe any signs or symptoms that concern you—for example, discharge, itching, painful intercourse, sores, fever, chills, or swelling? If the patient has specific complaints, ask her questions about the onset, duration, and severity of the problem. Also find out what precipitates the symptom, what makes it worse, and what makes it better.

Reproductive health

☐ How old were you when you began menstruating?

☐ When was the first day of your last menstrual period?

☐ Was that menstrual period normal compared with previous menstrual periods?

☐ How often do you menstruate? For how long?

☐ How would you describe your menstrual flow? For example, how many pads or tampons do you use on each day?

☐ Before your menstrual period begins, do you experience such changes as headaches, weight gain, swelling, breast tenderness, irritability, or mood swings? Do these changes occur with each menstrual period?

☐ Do you have pain or cramping during your menstrual periods? If so, how would you describe the discomfort? How long does it usually last? Does it interfere with your ability to perform your usual activities? How do you treat this problem?

☐ Have you stopped menstruating? If so, how do you account for the cessation?

☐ Do you have any symptoms of menopause, such as hot flashes, flushing, or mood swings? What are your feelings about going through menopause?

☐ Do you ever bleed between menstrual periods? If so, how much do you bleed and for how long?

☐ Do you ever have vaginal bleeding after intercourse?

☐ Has anyone ever told you that something is different about your uterus or other reproductive organs?

☐ When was your last Papanicolaou (Pap) test? Have you ever had a positive Pap test?

☐ Have you had surgery for a reproductive problem?

☐ Do you practice contraception?

☐ Do you use an oral contraceptive or another type of contraceptive? How long have you used a contraceptive? If it's a device, is it in good condition?

☐ Have you ever been pregnant?

☐ Have you ever had difficulty conceiving?

☐ Have you ever had an abortion or miscarriage?

☐ How many children have you had? Were they delivered vaginally or surgically?

Sexual-social health

☐ Are your sexual practices bisexual, homosexual, or heterosexual?

☐ Are you currently sexually active? If so, when did you last have sexual intercourse?

☐ Are you sexually active with more than one partner?

☐ Have you ever had a sexually transmitted disease (STD) or a genital infection?

☐ Are you satisfied with communication between you and your partner about your sexual needs?

☐ Does your sexual partner have any signs or symptoms of infection, such as genital sores, warts, or discharge?

☐ Have you ever been sexually active with anyone who uses I.V. drugs or is otherwise at risk for carrying and transmitting the human immunodeficiency virus (HIV) that causes acquired immunodeficiency syndrome?

☐ Have you ever been tested for HIV infection? What do you do to reduce the risk of contracting HIV and other STDs?

Family health

☐ Has anyone in your family ever had reproductive problems or gynecologic surgery?

☐ Has anyone in your family ever had twins?

☐ Has anyone in your family ever had diabetes, hypertension, obesity, or cancer of the reproductive organs?

General health

☐ What drugs (for example, prescription, nonprescription, illicit) are you currently taking? How often do you take them, at what dosage, and why?

☐ Do you drink alcoholic beverages? If so, how much do you drink? How long have you been drinking?

☐ Do you smoke? If so, how much do you smoke? How long have you smoked?

Preparing for the assessment

To begin, obtain two pairs of clean gloves, water-soluble lubricant, tissues, and a drape or blanket. You'll also need access to running water.

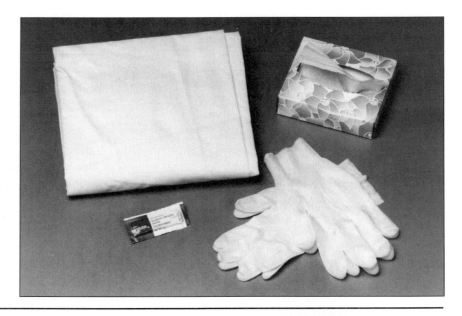

Before the examination, ask the patient to urinate because a full bladder produces discomfort and interferes with accurate palpation. Then ask her to remove all her clothing (except for her socks) and put on a disposable gown.

Assist the patient into the lithotomy position on the examination table. The table should have stirrups or knee supports. Place the patient's legs so that her feet or knees are appropriately positioned in the apparatus. Adjust the stirrups or knee supports so that her legs are comfortably separated.

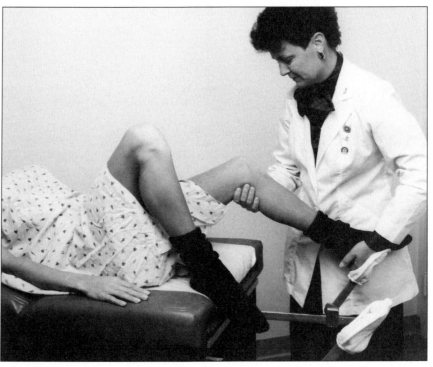

Once the patient's legs and feet are positioned correctly, help her slide to the lower edge of the examination table until her buttocks rest on the edge of the table.

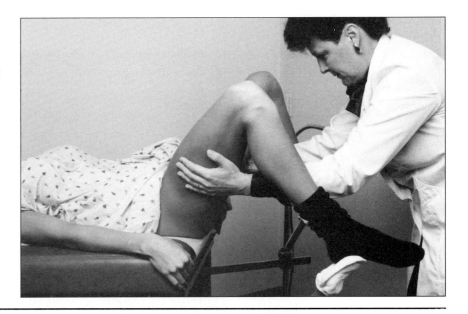

Place the drape over the patient's abdomen and knees. To help her relax her abdominal muscles, put a small pillow under her head. Have her place her arms at her sides.

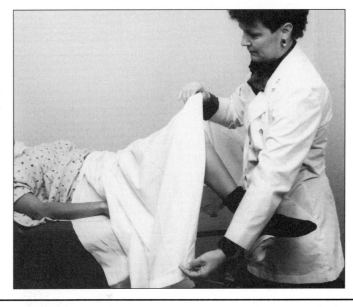

Position your stool at the foot of the table between the patient's legs. Adjust the light source so that it shines on the draped genital area. Explain the examination steps to the patient, and describe what she will feel.

▶ *Clinical tip:* Inform the patient that tightening her lower vaginal wall during the examination is a normal reflex. Instruct her to relax by inhaling slowly and deeply through the nose, exhaling through the mouth, and concentrating on breathing regularly. A ceiling poster or mobile may also help to distract her.

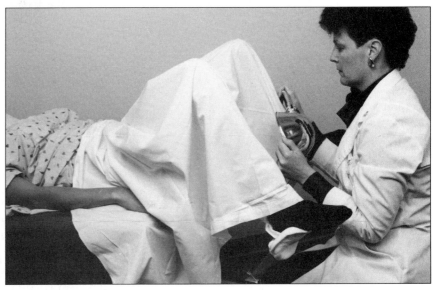

Sit on the stool at the foot of the examination table, and adjust the height of the drape between the patient's legs so that you can maintain eye contact with her. Wash your hands and put on the two pairs of examination gloves. Make sure that the examination equipment is on a movable table within easy reach.

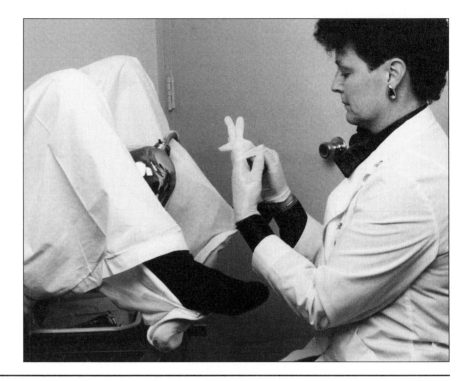

Inspecting the external genitalia

Begin by observing the external genitalia and the pubic hair to assess sexual maturity. Also inspect the labia majora, spreading the hair to check for lesions, parasites, and genital warts. Expect the skin to be slightly darker than the rest of the body. The labia majora should be round and full.

▶ *Clinical tip:* Use the patient's pubic hair characteristics as a guide to sexual maturity. Pubic hair changes in density, color, and texture throughout a person's lifespan. In preadolescence, the female has only body hair. In adolescence, the hair grows thicker, darker, coarser, and curlier. In full maturity, it spreads over the symphysis pubis and inner thighs. In later years, the hair grows thin, gray, and brittle.

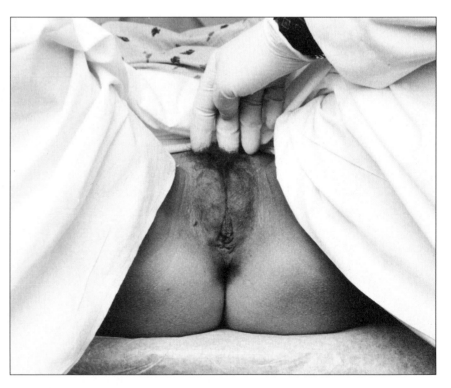

Using a gloved index finger and thumb, gently spread the labia majora and examine them and the labia minora. The latter should be moist and lesion-free. You may detect a normal cervical discharge varying from clear and stretchy before ovulation to white and opaque after ovulation. The discharge is usually odorless and nonirritating to the mucosa.

Examine the vestibule, especially the area around Bartholin's and Skene's glands. Look for swelling, redness, lesions, or discharge. If you notice any lesions, abnormal discharge, or unusual odor, notify the doctor, and obtain a specimen for culture.

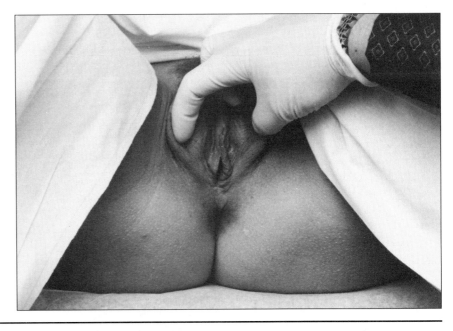

Inspect the urethral opening. It should be slitlike and the same color as the mucous membranes. Look for erythema, polyps, or discharge.

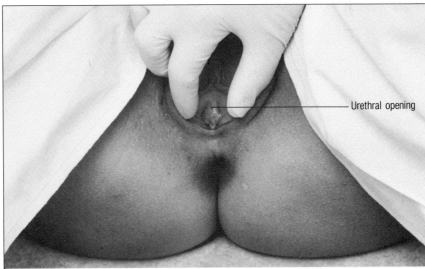

Urethral opening

Inspect the vaginal opening. It will be a thin vertical slit in a woman with an intact hymen and a large opening with irregular edges in a woman with a perforated hymen.

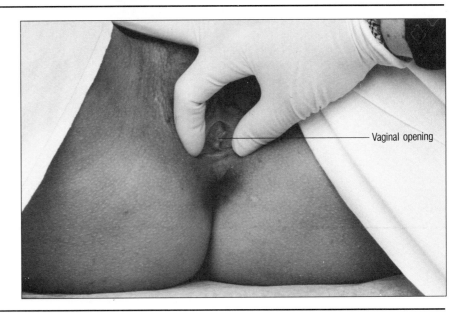

Vaginal opening

Palpating the external genitalia

Spread the labia open with one hand as you palpate them with your other hand. They should feel soft. Note any swelling, hardness, or tenderness. If you detect a mass or lesion, palpate it to determine its size, shape, and consistency.

If you find labial swelling or tenderness, palpate the area of Bartholin's glands (which aren't normally palpable). Insert your gloved index finger into the patient's posterior introitus, and place your thumb along the lateral edge of the swollen or tender labium. If appropriate, obtain a specimen of any discharge for culture.

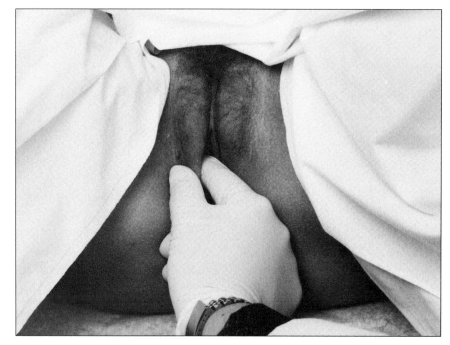

If you note urethral inflammation, milk the urethra and the area of Skene's glands. First, moisten your gloved index finger with water. Separate the labia with your other gloved hand, and gently insert your index finger about 1¼" (4 cm) into the anterior vagina. With your finger pad, gently press and pull outward. Continue palpating down to the introitus (as shown).

This procedure should not cause discomfort. Obtain a specimen of any discharge for culture, if appropriate.

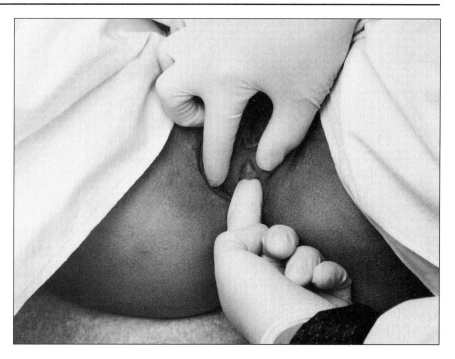

Inspecting the internal genitalia

Select a speculum that's appropriate for the patient—usually a Graves speculum. However, if the patient has an intact hymen, has never given birth, or has a contracted introitus from menopause, use a Pederson speculum.

Hold the speculum under warm running water to lubricate and warm the blades. If you're using a plastic speculum, explain that it may make a clicking sound when the blades move.

▶ *Clinical tip:* Avoid placing commercial lubricants on the speculum blades because these preparations are bacteriostatic. They'll alter Pap test and culture results.

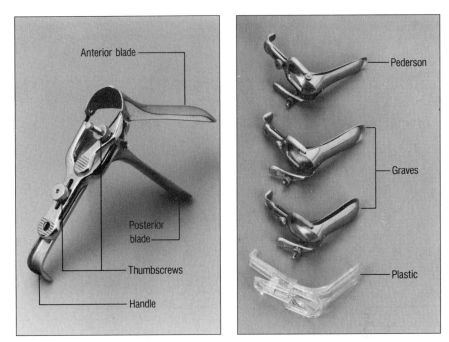

Sit or stand at the foot of the examination table. Tell the patient to expect some internal pressure as you insert and open the speculum. Using your dominant hand, hold the speculum by the base with the blades anchored between your index and middle fingers. This will keep the blades from accidentally opening during insertion.

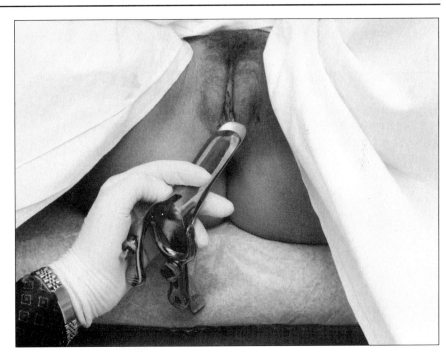

Insert the middle and index fingers of your other hand about 1″ (2.5 cm) into the vagina and spread them apart, pressing downward to put pressure on the posterior vagina. Hold the speculum sideways with the handle at a 45-degree angle between the patient's legs and the floor. Then insert the speculum between your fingers.

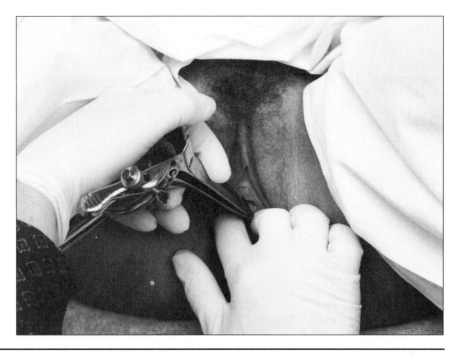

As you insert the speculum, rotate it until the handle points to the floor and the blades are parallel to the floor. While turning the speculum, withdraw your fingers from the vagina.

▶ *Clinical tip:* Remind the patient to take slow deep breaths to relax her abdominal muscles. Reassure her that any discomfort is transient.

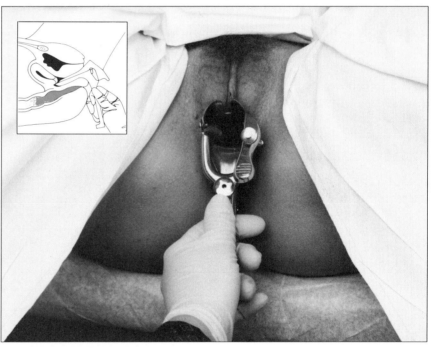

You can also use your other hand to help insert the blades farther into the vagina (as shown). As you insert the speculum, observe the color, texture, and integrity of the vaginal lining. A thin, white, odorless discharge is normal.

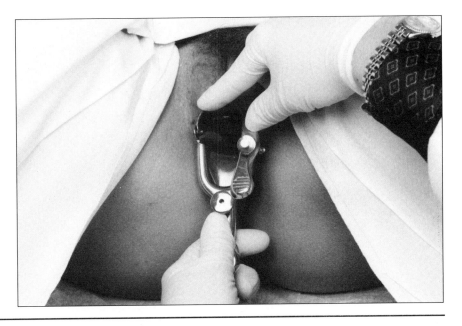

Using the thumb of the hand holding the speculum, press the lower lever to open the blades. Then lock them in the open position by tightening the thumbscrew above the lever (as shown).

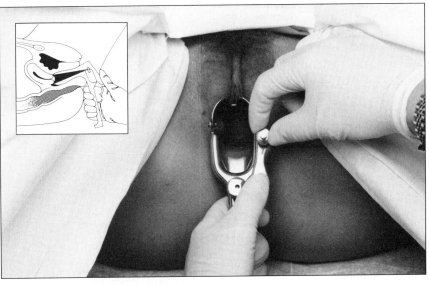

Examine the cervix for color, position, size, shape, mucosal integrity, and discharge. It should be smooth and round. The central cervical opening (the cervical os) is circular in a woman who hasn't given birth vaginally and stellate or star-shaped in a woman who has.

Expect to see a clear, watery discharge during ovulation or a slightly bloody discharge just before menstruation. Obtain a specimen for culture if you observe any other discharge. Use the spatula to obtain a specimen for a Pap test.

Finally, unlock and close the blades to withdraw the speculum.

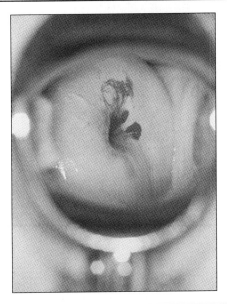

Palpating the internal genitalia

Stand at the foot of the examination table. Then lubricate the index and middle fingers of your dominant hand, and position this hand for insertion into the vagina by extending your thumb, index, and middle fingers, and curling your ring and little fingers toward your palm.

Use the thumb and index finger of your other hand to spread the labia majora. Insert the lubricated fingers into the vagina, exerting pressure posteriorly to avoid irritating the anterior wall and urethra.

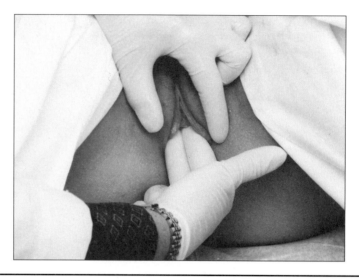

When your fingers are fully inserted in the vagina, note any tenderness or nodularity in the vaginal wall.

Note: Although the patient would normally be draped, the drape has been removed here and in the following photographs to provide an unobstructed view.

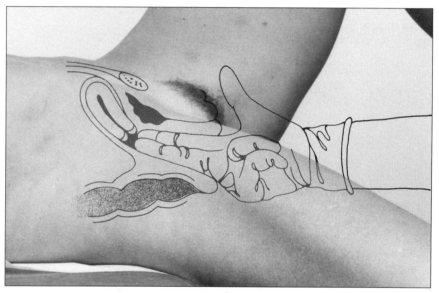

Palpate the urethra by sweeping your fingers along the anterior vaginal wall toward the vaginal opening. Expect the urethra to feel soft and tubular. Note any discharge or tenderness.

Ask the patient to bear down so that you can assess the support of the vaginal outlet. Bulging of the vaginal wall may indicate a cystocele or a rectocele.

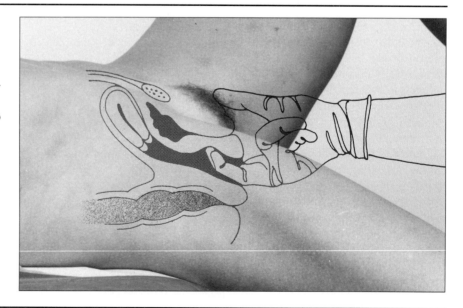

Ask the patient to relax as you palpate the cervix. Sweep your fingers from side to side across the cervix and around the os. Expect the cervix to be smooth and firm and to protrude ½″ to 1¼″ (1 to 3 cm) into the vagina. If you palpate nodules or irregularities, suspect cysts, tumors, or other lesions.

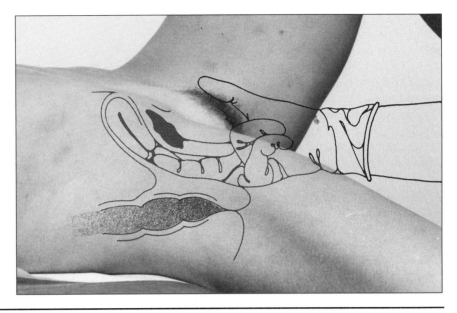

Place your fingers into the recessed area around the cervix (the fornix) and gently move the cervix. The cervix should move ½″ to ¾″ (1 to 2 cm) in any direction. If the patient reports pain during this part of the examination, she may have a uterine or adnexal inflammation.

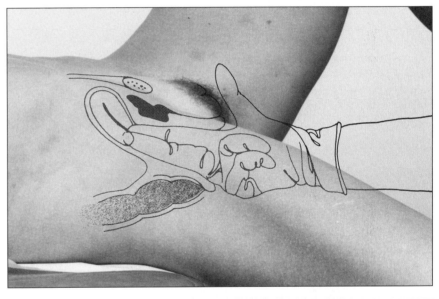

Place your free hand on the patient's abdomen between the umbilicus and the symphysis pubis. Elevate the cervix and uterus by pressing upward with the two fingers inside the vagina. At the same time, press down and in with the hand on the abdomen. Try to grasp the uterus between your hands.

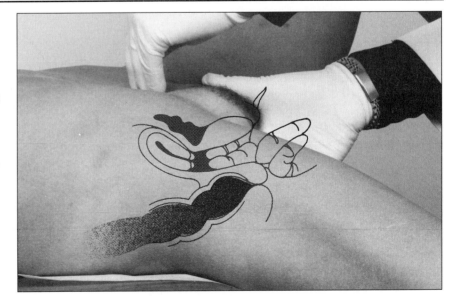

Slide your fingers farther into the anterior section of the fornix. Expect to feel part of the posterior uterine wall with your nondominant hand (the hand pressing into the abdomen). Expect the fingertips of your dominant hand to feel part of the anterior uterine wall.

Note the size, shape, surface characteristics, consistency, mobility, and any tenderness of the uterus.

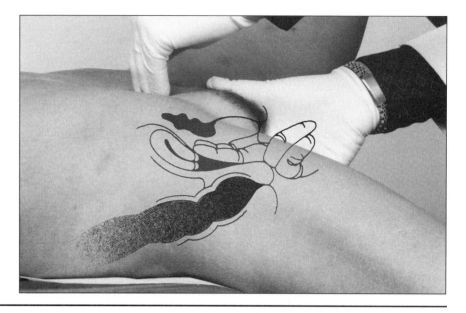

Move your fingers into the posterior fornix, pressing upward and forward to bring the anterior uterine wall up to your nondominant hand. Use your dominant hand to palpate the lower portion of the uterine wall. Note the position of the uterus.

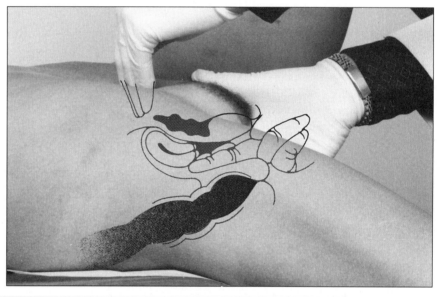

Move your nondominant hand toward the right lower quadrant. Slip the fingers of your dominant hand into the right fornix and palpate the right ovary. Note its size (normally 1¼" to 1½", or 3 to 4 cm), shape (ovoid), and contour (flat). Then palpate the left ovary.

Remove your hand from the patient's abdomen and your fingers from her vagina. Discard your outer pair of gloves.

▶ *Clinical tip:* Usually, you can palpate the ovaries in a premenopausal woman but not in a menopausal woman. If you can, suspect an abnormality, such as an ovarian tumor.

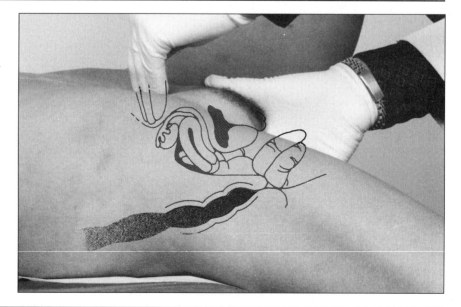

Palpating the rectovaginal area

To complete the genital assessment, examine the rectal structures adjoining the vaginal area. Forewarn the patient that this final part of the examination may cause some discomfort.

Then apply water-soluble lubricant to the index and middle fingers of your gloved dominant hand. Instruct the patient to bear down with her vaginal and rectal muscles. As she does, insert your index finger slightly into her vagina and your middle finger into her rectum. Use your middle finger to assess rectal muscle and sphincter tone.

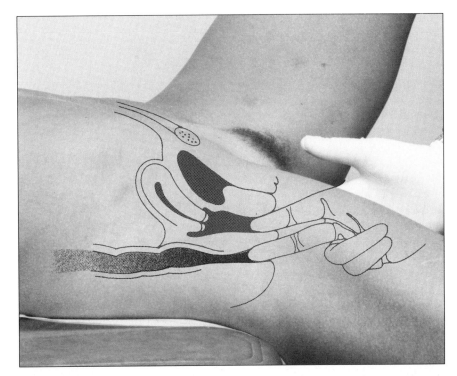

Insert your fingers deeper and palpate the patient's rectal wall with your middle finger. The rectovaginal septum—the wall between the rectum and the vagina—should feel smooth and springy. When your fingers are fully inserted, gently squeeze the rectovaginal septum. This structure should be free of masses, deviations, and tenderness.

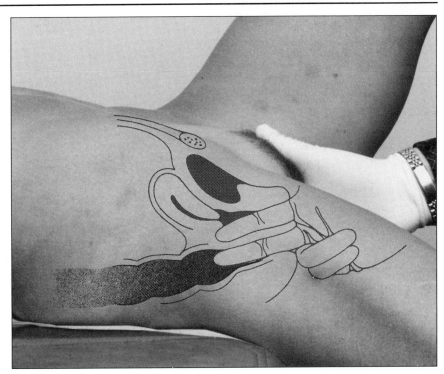

Place your nondominant hand on the patient's abdomen at the symphysis pubis. Palpate deeply to feel the posterior edge of the cervix and the lower posterior wall of the uterus (with the index finger in the vagina).

At the same time, palpate the upper posterior wall of the uterus through the rectal wall (with the middle finger in the rectum). Palpate for masses, deviations, and tenderness. Probe deeply with your fingertips to locate the pouch of Douglas. This action should not elicit tenderness.

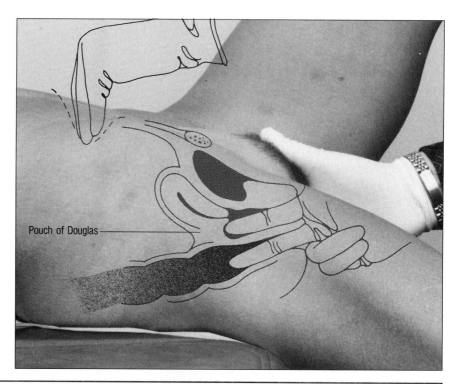

Withdraw your fingers, discard your gloves, and wash your hands. Assist the patient to a sitting position. Offer her a tissue to remove remaining lubricant. Document the procedure.

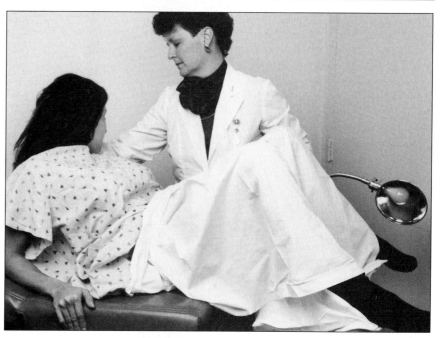

Identifying uterine positions

The normal uterus usually tips slightly forward, though this may vary, depending on the fullness of the bladder. Several other uterine positions can be palpated during a bimanual examination. In the chart below, external findings refer to external palpation of the abdomen and internal findings refer to palpation through the vagina. Uterine position can affect fertility or signal a disorder.

POSITION		EXTERNAL FINDINGS	INTERNAL FINDINGS	RECTOVAGINAL FINDINGS
Normal Uterus tipped forward slightly above bladder—almost at 90-degree angle to cervix; cervix tipped downward	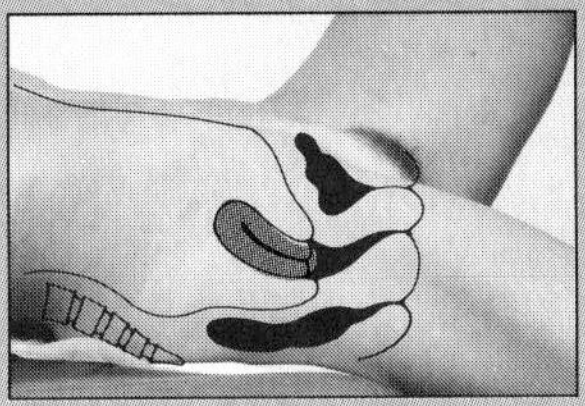	• Up to one-quarter of posterior uterine wall palpable • Up to one-half of anterior uterine wall palpable	• Up to three-quarters of anterior uterine wall palpable • Up to one-half of lower posterior uterine wall palpable in posterior fornix	• Pouch of Douglas palpable • Posterior uterine wall palpable
Midposition Uterus nearly vertical on same plane as cervix, which points straight forward	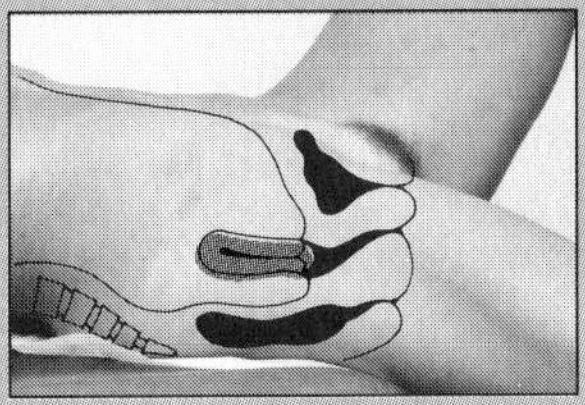	• Fingers in anterior fornix palpable • Uterine wall usually not palpable	• Fingers on abdomen palpable • Lower one-quarter of posterior uterine wall palpable in posterior fornix • Lower one-quarter of anterior uterine wall palpable with downward pressure in anterior fornix	• Posterior edge of cervix palpable • Pouch of Douglas palpable
Anteflexed Body of uterus tipped forward at 90-degree angle to cervix, which tips downward	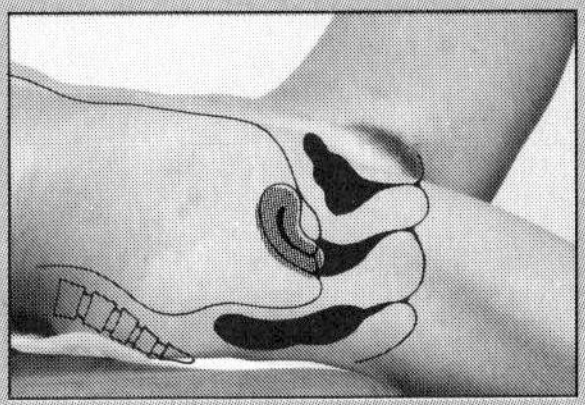	• Upper one-half of posterior uterine wall palpable	• Up to one-half of posterior uterine wall palpable • Uterine fundus palpable in anterior fornix • Anterior uterine wall not palpable • In extreme anteflexion, fingers on abdomen palpable	• Small portion of posterior cervix palpable • Pouch of Douglas palpable
Anteverted Uterus tipped forward on same plane as cervix, which tips downward	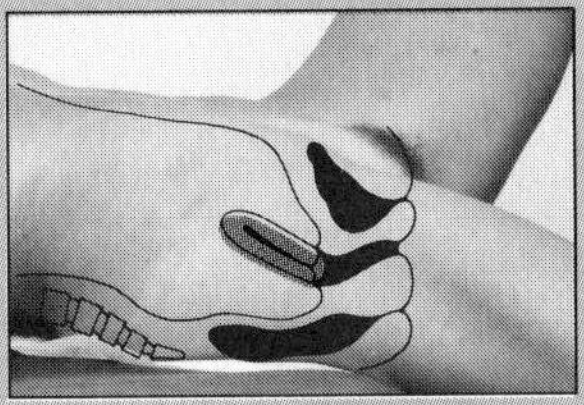	• Up to one-half of anterior uterine wall palpable • Upper one-quarter of posterior fundus palpable	• Up to three-quarters of lower anterior uterine wall palpable • Up to one-half of lower posterior uterine wall palpable in posterior fornix	• Posterior edge of cervix palpable • Pouch of Douglas palpable
Retroflexed Body of uterus tipped backward at 90-degree angle to cervix, which tips upward	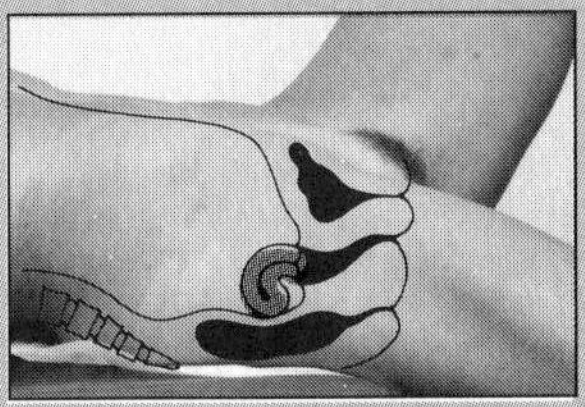	• Fingers in anterior fornix palpable • Lower one-quarter of anterior uterine wall palpable	• Lower one-quarter of anterior uterine wall palpable • Uterine fundus palpable in posterior fornix	• Up to one-half of anterior uterine wall and posterior cervical wall palpable
Retroverted Uterus tipped backward on same plane as cervix, which tips upward	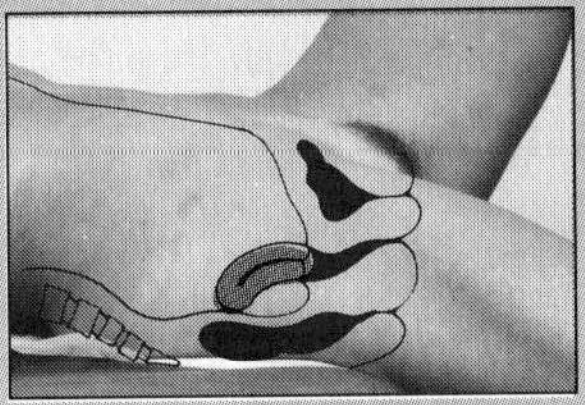	• Fingers in anterior fornix palpable • Uterine wall not palpable	• Anterior and lower portion of anterior uterine wall palpable • Lower one-half of posterior uterine wall palpable in posterior fornix	• Portion of posterior cervix palpable • Pouch of Douglas palpable • Lower one-quarter of anterior and posterior uterine wall palpable

EXAMINING THE MALE GENITALIA

You'll need to understand the patient's anatomy and its function to accurately assess his reproductive health. (See *Anatomy of the male reproductive system.*) A main part of the assessment will be a thorough genital and reproductive health history (see *Exploring male reproductive health complaints*) and an emphasis on health maintenance and disease prevention. (See the patient-teaching aid *How to examine your testicles,* page 146.)

Anatomy of the male reproductive system

The male genitalia include the penis, scrotum and testicles, epididymis and vas deferens, seminal vesicles, and prostate gland.

Penis
Consisting of a shaft, glans, corona, and urethral meatus, the penis is the main reproductive organ. The shaft consists of vascular erectile tissue, which encases the urethra. The glans at the end of the penis has a slitlike opening—the urethral meatus. The corona is a ridge of tissue formed by the junction of the glans and the shaft. The prepuce (or foreskin), which loosely covers the glans, is commonly removed soon after birth by circumcision.

Scrotum and testicles
At the base of the penis, the scrotum consists of muscle covered by a thin layer of skin. It divides into two compartments, each containing a testicle and branches of the spermatic cord. The spermatic cord passes up through the abdominal muscle via the inguinal canal. The external opening of the inguinal canal is a triangular slitlike structure, palpable on physical examination. The testicles—rubbery, ovate structures—are suspended in the scrotum. These glands produce testosterone and sperm.

Seminal vesicles and prostate gland
The seminal vesicles lie on the bladder's surface in front of the rectum. The prostate, a walnut-shaped gland about 2½″ (6 cm) long, surrounds the urethra just below the bladder. The seminal vesicles and the prostate secrete fluids that mix with sperm at ejaculation, enhance spermatic motility, and increase the chance of fertilization.

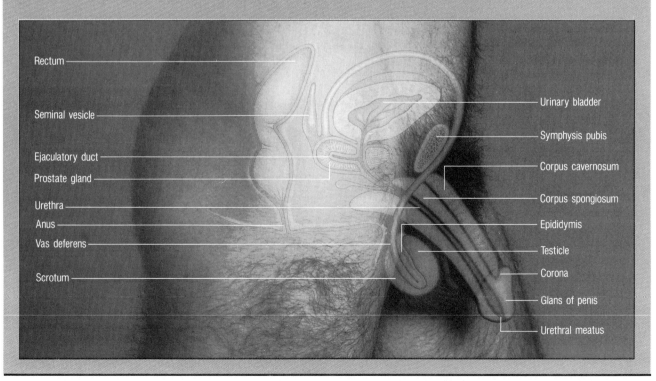

Rectum

Seminal vesicle

Ejaculatory duct

Prostate gland

Urethra

Anus

Vas deferens

Scrotum

Urinary bladder

Symphysis pubis

Corpus cavernosum

Corpus spongiosum

Epididymis

Testicle

Corona

Glans of penis

Urethral meatus

ASSESSMENT CHECKLIST

Exploring male reproductive health complaints

To fully evaluate your patient's reproductive health status, obtain a complete history focused on his current complaint and his genitourinary, reproductive, sexual-social, family, and general health. Ask questions such as the ones in this checklist.

Current complaint

☐ What brought you in for an examination today? (Guide the patient with more specific questions if he has trouble identifying a single complaint.)

☐ Can you describe any signs or symptoms that concern you (such as changes in the color of the penile or the scrotal skin)?

☐ Are you circumcised? If not, can you retract and replace your foreskin (prepuce) easily?

☐ Do you have any sores or masses on your penis?

☐ Have you noticed any discharge or bleeding from your penis?

☐ Have you noticed any swelling in your scrotum?

☐ Are you experiencing any pain in the penis, testicles, or scrotum? Does the pain radiate? If so, where? When does it occur? What measures aggravate or relieve the pain?

☐ Have you felt a mass, a painful sore, or tenderness in your groin?

Genitourinary health

☐ Do you get up during the night to urinate? Do you have frequent or hesitant urination or dribbling? Do you have pain in the area between your rectum and penis? Do you have pain in your hips or lower back?

☐ Have you ever had genitourinary surgery? If so, where, when, and why? Did you have complications?

☐ Have you ever had a genitourinary injury? If so, what happened, when did it occur, and what, if any, residual symptoms or problems do you have?

☐ Have you ever had blood in your urine, difficulty urinating, an excessive urge to urinate, dribbling, or difficulty maintaining the urine stream?

☐ Do you or did you have undescended testicles or an endocrine disorder? Have you ever had mumps? If so, did the disease affect your testicles?

☐ Do you examine your testicles periodically? Have you been taught the proper procedure?

Reproductive health

☐ Have you fathered any children? If so, how many?

☐ Have you ever had a problem with infertility or a low sperm count? Is this a current concern?

☐ What kind of work do you do? Are you now or have you ever been exposed to radiation or toxic chemicals?

☐ Do you engage in sports or activities that require lifting heavy objects or straining? If so, do you wear any protective or supportive devices?

Sexual-social health

☐ Are your sexual practices homosexual, bisexual, or heterosexual?

☐ Are you sexually active? Do you have more than one partner? How many partners have you had during the last month?

☐ Do you have any difficulty achieving and maintaining an erection during sexual activity? Do you have erections at other times, such as on awakening?

☐ Do you have any difficulty with ejaculation?

☐ Do you ever experience pain from erection or ejaculation?

☐ Are you under a lot of stress?

☐ If you're having sexual difficulty, is it affecting your relationships or interfering with your daily life?

☐ Have you ever been diagnosed as having a sexually transmitted disease (STD) or any other infection in the genitourinary tract? If so, what was the specific problem? How long did it last? What treatment was provided? Did complications develop?

☐ Have you ever been tested for the human immunodeficiency virus (HIV), the organism that causes acquired immunodeficiency syndrome (AIDS)?

☐ Have you ever had a sexual encounter with anyone with HIV or anyone at risk for HIV?

☐ What precautions do you take to prevent contracting an STD or AIDS?

Family health

☐ Has anyone in your family had infertility problems or a hernia?

☐ Has anyone in your family had cancer of the reproductive tract?

General health

☐ Have you had diabetes mellitus, cardiovascular disease, neurologic disease, or cancer of the genitourinary tract?

☐ What drugs (prescription, nonprescription, or illicit) do you take? At what dosage and for what reason? How long have you taken them?

☐ Do you drink alcohol? If so, how much do you drink? How long have you been drinking?

Preparing for the genital assessment

Begin the physical examination by gathering the necessary equipment, including several pairs of gloves, water-soluble lubricant, and tissues. Have hemoculture slides and developer available in case you need to obtain a specimen for culture or analysis.

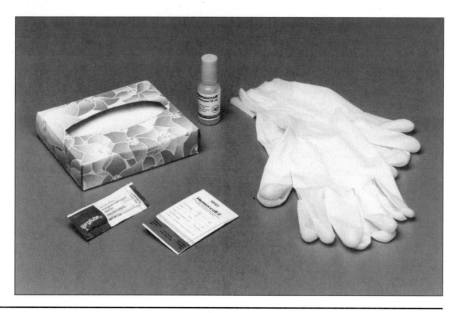

Inspecting and palpating the pelvis and groin

Wash your hands, put on gloves, and explain the examination to the patient. Ask him to urinate and to disrobe from the waist down. Offer him a gown or a drape for privacy. Then ask him to stand facing you. (If he can't stand, have him lie on his back on an examination table.)

Observe the patient's pelvis, which should be symmetrical and triangular. Note the amount and characteristics of pubic hair, and look for any discolorations or masses. Carefully inspect the groin area (indicated by the shading). This is where hernias may occur.

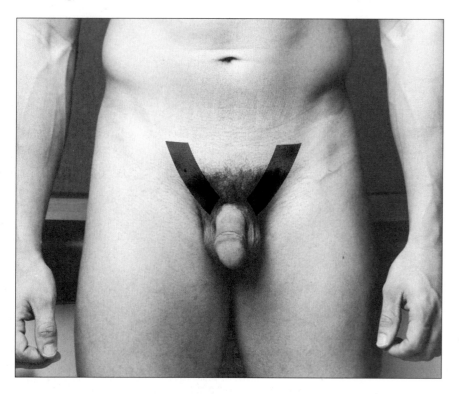

Ask the patient to hold his penis off to his left. Then, using your index and middle fingers, palpate his right inguinal area for masses or bulges. Ask the patient to bear down as you continue to palpate for abnormalities, especially a sliding sensation against your fingertips.

▶ *Clinical tip:* Use your right hand to palpate the patient's right groin and your left hand to palpate his left groin.

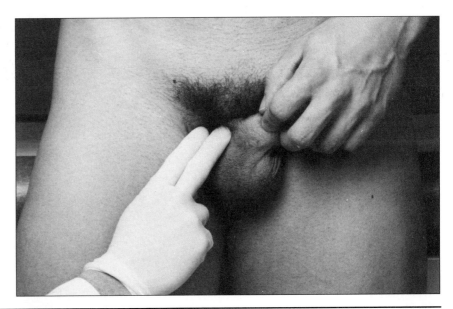

To examine the patient's right inguinal ring, place your right index finger on the scrotum, slightly below and to the right of the penis (as shown).

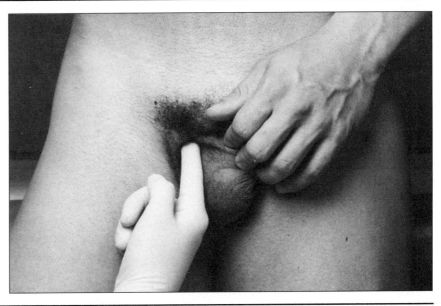

Gently push upward at a 45-degree angle to infold the loose scrotal skin. As you do so, insert your finger farther so that it passes into the patient's inguinal area along the path of the spermatic cord. When your finger is fully inserted, you should feel the pubic bone with your fingertip (as shown).

▶ *Clinical tip:* Be careful not to pinch the skin of the scrotum or the spermatic cord because this will be painful to the patient.

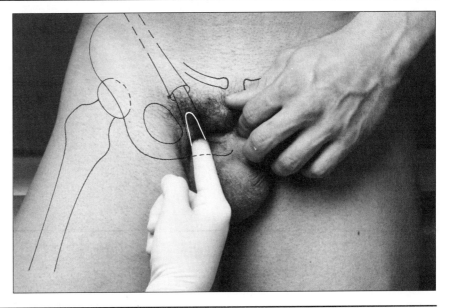

Next, move your finger about ½″ (1 cm) above and lateral to the pubic bone's edge, and palpate the triangular opening of the external inguinal ring. Expect the ring to be unobstructed. A mass that protrudes through the inguinal ring suggests an inguinal hernia. In this case, tell the patient to bear down and cough.

If inner tissue slides against your fingertip, suspect a hernia above the inguinal ring. If the tissue strikes the side of your finger, suspect a direct hernia. If the tissue strikes your fingertip, suspect an indirect hernia. Reverse the procedure to examine the patient's other side.

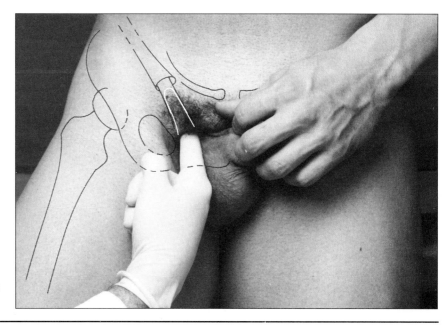

Inspecting and palpating the penis

Explain this procedure before continuing. Observe the patient's penis. In a circumcised patient, the glans will be exposed above a ridge of tissue (the corona) at the base (near right). In an uncircumcised patient, a foreskin (the prepuce) will cover the glans (far right).

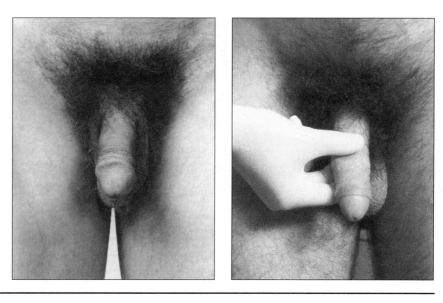

Lift the penis to examine the posterior surface. Expect it to be smooth without ulcers, swelling, scars, discolorations, or nodules. Feel for abnormalities with your index and middle fingers.

In an uncircumcised patient, place your thumb and index finger on either side of the foreskin and gently retract the foreskin over the penile shaft. If the foreskin fails to slide easily, the patient may have phimosis. If the foreskin is constricted behind the glans, he may have paraphimosis.

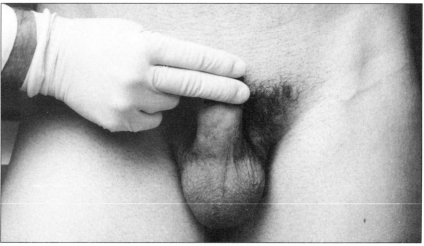

Hold the shaft of the penis and examine the glans (near right). Expect it to be smooth and cone shaped. Note any lesions, hardened areas, growths, swelling, inflammation, or discoloration. Expect the urethral meatus to be at the tip of the penis. If it's not there, document its exact location.

Place your thumbs on either side of the urinary meatus, and gently move them outward to open the meatus (far right). Look for lesions, strictures, or discharge. If appropriate, obtain a specimen for culture. In an uncircumcised patient, gently replace the foreskin.

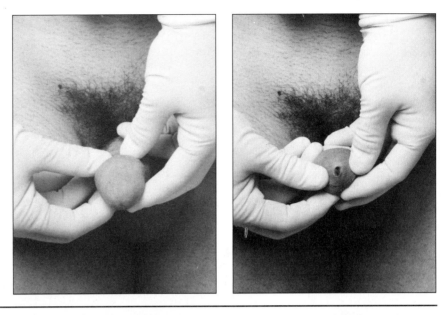

To palpate the penile shaft, place the thumb and index fingers of both hands at the base of the penis. Position your fingers to cover as much of the surface as you can.

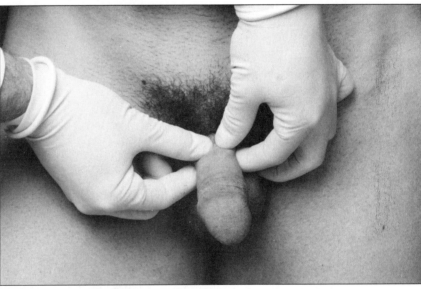

Then slide your fingers down the shaft to the base of the glans. As you move your fingers, rotate them slightly from side to side to palpate the entire penis.

Expect a healthy adult penis to feel soft but not flabby. (In an older patient, the penis may be slightly flabby.) Be alert for thickening, nodules, protrusions, or hardness.

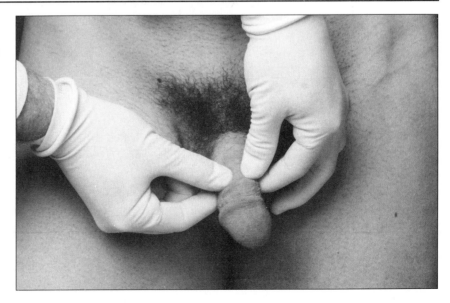

Inspecting and palpating the scrotum

Before continuing, explain scrotal examination to the patient. Then lift the penis up and against the symphysis pubis to assess the scrotum (near right). Normally, the scrotal sac appears almost symmetrical, with the left side hanging slightly lower. Expect the scrotal skin to be wrinkled but to firmly hug the testicles.

Lift the scrotal sac up to inspect the posterior surface (far right). Note any swelling, nodules, inflammation, ulcers, or distended veins.

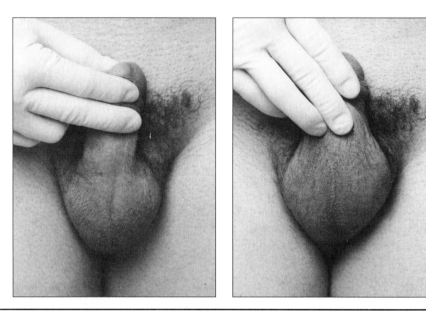

To palpate the scrotum, hold the penis up out of the way and place your index finger on the posterior surface and your thumb on the anterior surface. Move your fingers to the right, and gently press them together. The patient may report slight tenderness. If a testicle isn't palpable, it may have migrated.

▶ *Clinical tip:* Be careful to distinguish between a congenitally undescended testicle and one that has migrated toward the inguinal canal in response to such stimuli as touch and cold.

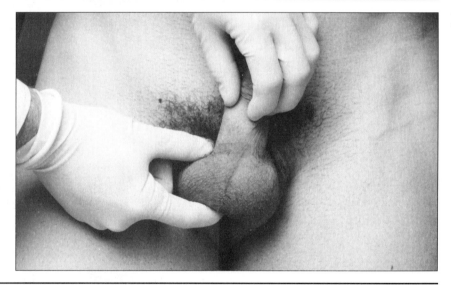

Move your fingers to the left and palpate the left testicle (as shown). Both testicles should be similar in size, shape, and consistency. Palpate the epididymis, a small ridge of tissue lying vertically on the surface of the testicle.

If you detect a mass in the epididymis or elsewhere in the scrotum, try to press your fingers together above it. If your fingers meet, the mass is probably contained in the scrotum. If they don't meet, the mass may extend downward from the abdomen.

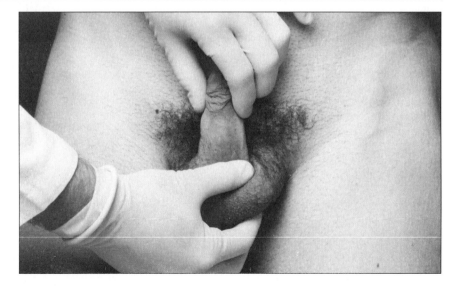

Locate the spermatic cord for palpation by sliding your thumb and index finger to the top of the testicle. Expect to feel a smooth, round cordlike structure extending from the top of the testicle. It should be firm and bouncy.

A soft, movable mass along the cord may be an accumulation of fluid (or hydrocele). A group of hard, nodular, cordlike structures along the cord may indicate varicoceles, varices, or varicose veins.

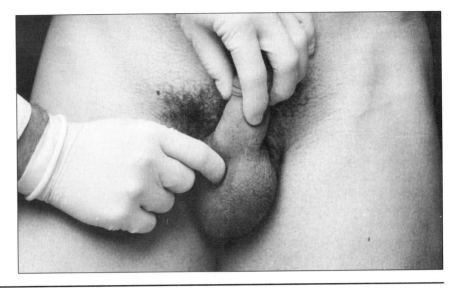

Inspecting and palpating the rectum, prostate gland, and seminal vesicles

As always, explain the procedure. Ask the patient to face the examination table and bend over so that his upper body rests on the table. (If the patient can't stand, have him lie on his left side at the edge of the table and bend his knees toward his chest.)

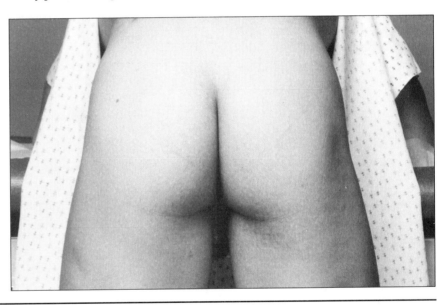

Inspect the patient's buttocks by gently pushing both buttocks outward with your hands. Examine the area between his buttocks for masses, inflammation, or skin tears. The anal opening should appear puckered and dark.

Instruct the patient to bear down. Observe the anal opening for protrusions. Reddish protrusions made up of distended veins indicate hemorrhoids. Reddish velvety tissue projecting from the anus may indicate prolapsed rectal mucosa.

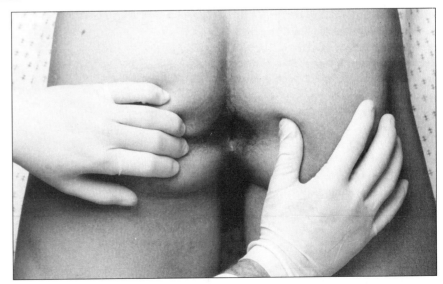

Apply water-soluble lubricant to the index finger of your dominant hand. Place your lubricated finger at the base of the patient's anal opening. Tell him to bear down. This will relax the anal sphincter.

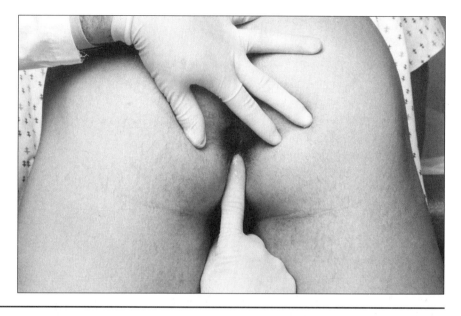

Gently slide your finger into the patient's anus up to the first joint of your finger. Note sphincter tone. Normally, it should feel tight—not flabby.

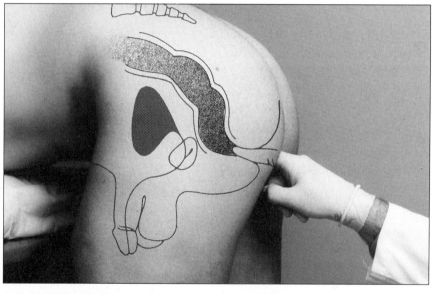

To palpate the anterior rectal wall, insert your finger deeper, and move it from side to side along the upper surface. Continue until you feel the prostate gland along the anterior wall about 2″ (5 cm) from the rectal opening. Warn the patient that he may feel a normal urge to urinate.

Expect the prostate to feel like a smooth, rubbery mass about 1¾″ (4 cm) in diameter and protruding into the rectum about ½″ (1 cm). Palpation shouldn't elicit tenderness.

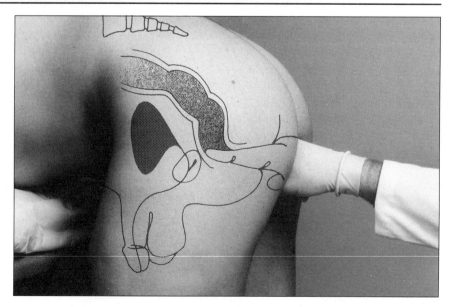

Extend your finger farther into the rectum and palpate the area of the seminal vesicles above the prostate gland. The seminal vesicles won't be palpable unless they are inflamed. Continue palpating as far in as your finger extends.

Rotate your hand until your palm faces up (as shown). Palpate the posterior rectal wall as you slide your finger out toward the anus. Note any masses, ulcers, or tenderness.

▶ *Clinical tip:* If you feel or suspect a mass just beyond your fingertip, ask the patient to bear down. This will bring any tissues at the tip of your fingers closer for a better examination.

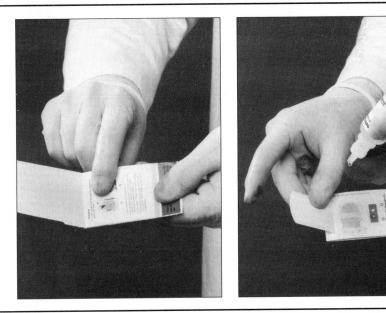

Remove your finger from the patient's rectum. Observe your finger for feces or traces of blood. If you see blood or if the doctor orders a hemoculture test, wipe your fingertip across a hemoculture slide (near right).

Drop several drops of developer on the specimen (far right), close the cover, label the slide, and send it to the laboratory. Then use a tissue to clean any remaining lubricant or fecal material from the patient's rectal area. Remove your gloves and wash your hands.

Put on new gloves. Tell the patient that to conclude the assessment, you need to reexamine the urinary meatus for any discharge caused by the rectal examination. Position your fingers (as shown) to again open the urinary meatus.

Normally, you should find no discharge. If you do, note this and obtain a discharge specimen for culture. Document your findings and any test procedures.

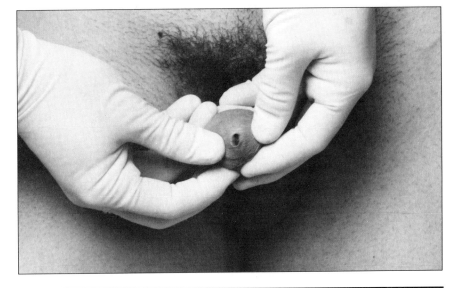

PATIENT TEACHING

How to examine your testicles

Dear Patient:

To detect testicular abnormalities at an early and treatable stage, examine yourself every month. The more familiar you are with your body, the easier it is to recognize any changes. Here's what to do:

1 If possible, first take a warm bath or shower. If the scrotum (the sac containing the testicles) stays warm, it's easier to examine.

Note: Some men find this examination easier to perform in front of a full-length mirror.

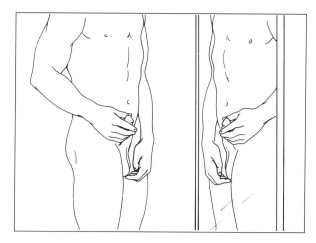

2 With one hand, lift the penis and check the scrotum for any change in shape, size, or color. Normally, the left side of the scrotum will hang slightly lower than the right side.

3 Next, check the testicles for masses. Locate the crescent-shaped structure at the back of each testicle. This is the epididymis; it should feel soft.

4 Use the thumb and first two fingers of your left hand to gently squeeze the spermatic cord (which extends upward from the epididymis above the left testicle). Re-

peat the procedure on the right side, using your right hand. Check for masses and changes by pressing along the entire length of the cord.

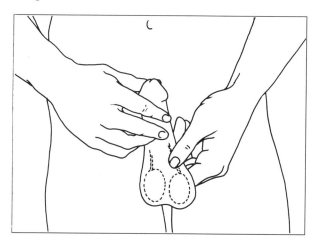

5 Next, examine each testicle. To do this, place your index and middle fingers of both hands on the underside of the testicle and your thumbs on top. Then gently roll the testicle between your thumb and fingers. A normal testicle is egg shaped, rubbery-firm, and movable within the scrotum. It should feel smooth and not lumpy. Both testicles should be the same size.

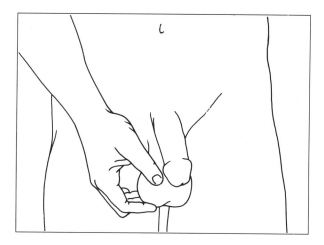

6 Promptly consult your doctor if you detect any masses or changes.

EXAMINING MUSCULOSKELETAL STRUCTURES

Composed of muscles, tendons, ligaments, and bones, the musculoskeletal system gives the human body form and mobility. The basic skeletal structure consists of 206 bones that support the body's organs and tissues, serve as storage sites for minerals, and produce red blood cells. (See *Bones of the skeletal system.*) Bones also unite to form joints (or articulations), which are held together by ligaments, and work in concert with the tendon-attached muscles to produce a

(continued)

Bones of the skeletal system

Of the 206 bones in the human skeletal system, 80 form the axial skeleton (the head and trunk) and 126 form the appendicular skeleton (the extremities). Featured below are the body's major bones.

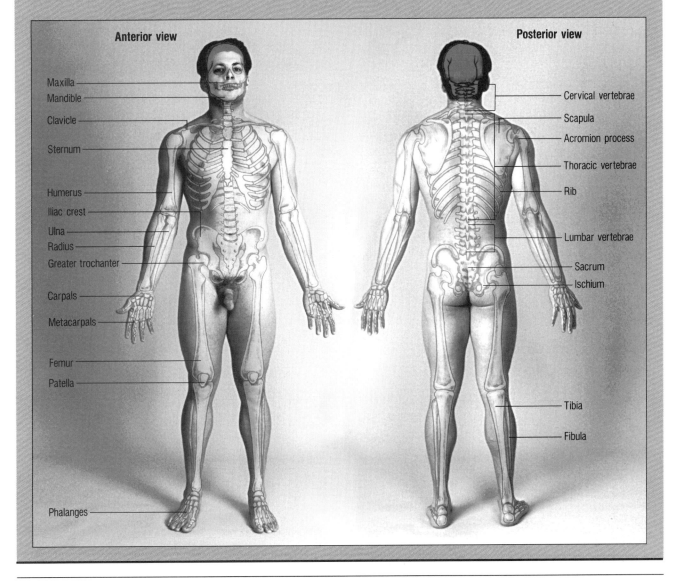

Anterior view

Maxilla
Mandible
Clavicle
Sternum
Humerus
Iliac crest
Ulna
Radius
Greater trochanter
Carpals
Metacarpals
Femur
Patella
Phalanges

Posterior view

Cervical vertebrae
Scapula
Acromion process
Thoracic vertebrae
Rib
Lumbar vertebrae
Sacrum
Ischium
Tibia
Fibula

Linda S. Baas, RN, PhD, CCRN, and *Brenda K. Shelton, RN, MS, CCRN, OCN,* contributed to this section. Ms. Baas is an assistant professor at the University of Cincinnati College of Nursing and Health. Ms. Shelton is a critical care clinical nurse specialist at The Johns Hopkins Oncology Center in Baltimore.

wide array of movements.

Of the various kinds of joints, many are stabilized by enclosure in a fibrous joint capsule. Each joint produces a predictable type of motion, which you'll assess in relation to the center of gravity for that part of the body (see *Body joints and range of motion*).

Composed of contractile cells or fibers, muscles trigger skeletal movement when stimulated by the central nervous system (CNS), which coordinates both voluntary and involuntary musculoskeletal function.

Because the CNS and the musculoskeletal system are intricately interrelated, you'll usually assess these systems simultaneously to prevent duplication of effort and patient fatigue.

MUSCULOSKELETAL ASSESSMENT

When you assess the musculoskeletal system, keep in mind that injury or inflammation of any part of the system can cause pain, stiffness, or an alteration in motor strength or mobility. Pay particular attention to the patient's health history and to complaints related to the musculoskeletal system. (See *Exploring musculoskeletal complaints*.)

In most cases, the musculoskeletal assessment progresses from head to toe with inspection, palpation, and range-of-motion (ROM) measurements.

Body joints and range of motion

Classified by the extent of movement they allow, joints are known as synarthrodial, amphidiarthrodial, or diarthrodial.

A synarthrodial joint separates bones with a thin layer of connective tissue, which allows no movement. An amphidiarthrodial joint connects adjacent bones with a hyaline cartilage, which permits slight movement. And a diarthrodial joint is a synovial membrane–lined cavity filled with a viscous lubricating fluid, which allows free movement. Joints are further identified by their shapes and characteristic motions.

TYPE OF JOINT	REPRESENTATIVE LOCATION	RANGE OF MOTION
Synarthrodial		
Suture	• Cranium (cranial suture)	Stationary
Synchondrosis	• Cranium • Sternum	No motion (a temporary cartilaginous juncture that precedes bone formation)
Amphidiarthrodial		
Symphysis	• Symphysis pubis	Slight motion because bones are joined with a fibrocartilaginous disk
Syndesmosis	• Radius and ulna • Tibia and fibula	Slight motion because bones are connected by ligaments
Diarthrodial		
Ball and socket	• Hip • Shoulder	Widest range of movement in all planes
Hinge	• Elbow	Limited to flexion and extension in a single plane
Pivot	• Atlantoaxial vertebrae (between first and second cervical vertebrae)	Limited to rotation
Condyloid	• Wrist, between the radius and the carpals	Limited to two planes at right angles to each other, without radial rotation
Saddle	• Thumb at carpal-metacarpal juncture	Limited to two planes at right angles to each other, without axial rotation
Gliding	• Spine (intervertebral)	Limited to gliding

Exploring musculoskeletal complaints

To pinpoint the source of your patient's musculoskeletal complaint, focus on specific problem areas. Here are some questions to guide your assessment of the patient's chief complaint, mobility, daily routine, and related medical history.

Chief complaint

☐ Are you having any pain or discomfort?

☐ Can you point to the painful area?

☐ How would you describe this pain or discomfort (for example, sharp, burning, aching, or throbbing)?

☐ Is your pain or discomfort limited to one area, or do you feel it in another area as well?

☐ When did this pain begin? What were you doing when it started?

☐ What activities decrease or eliminate the pain or discomfort?

☐ What activities increase or trigger the pain or discomfort?

☐ Do you have any other sensations along with the pain or discomfort (such as numbness or tingling)?

☐ Do you have any swelling, especially around a joint? If so, when did you first notice it?

☐ Did you injure the swollen area?

☐ Is the swollen area tender?

☐ Does the overlying skin ever appear red or feel hot?

☐ Have you tried to reduce the swelling or tenderness by using hot or cold packs?

☐ Do you take any prescription or nonprescription medications or home remedies to treat your problem? Describe these treatments and their effectiveness.

Mobility

☐ Do you have any stiffness? If so, does it interfere with movement?

☐ When did the stiffness begin? Has it increased?

☐ At what specific times do you feel stiff? Or do you feel stiff all the time?

☐ Does pain accompany the stiffness?

☐ What methods do you use to reduce the stiffness?

☐ Do you ever feel a grating sensation, like your bones are rubbing together?

☐ Do you hear a grating sound with movement?

☐ When did you first notice that your movement was impaired?

☐ Do you think that your movement is limited by stiffness or pain or something else? What else do you think may be causing the problem?

☐ Do you use an assistive device, such as a cane, walker, or brace? If not, do you think using such a device would help you?

Daily routine

☐ Have any of your usual activities, such as climbing stairs, rising from a chair, or driving, become difficult or impossible to do?

☐ Has your problem affected your job, hobbies or other leisure pursuits, or social life?

☐ Do you have problems with personal hygiene (for example, bathing, dressing, or grooming) because of pain, stiffness, or injury?

☐ Do you have trouble writing or feeding yourself?

☐ Do you have difficulty falling asleep?

☐ Does your problem cause you to wake up during the night?

☐ Do you follow an exercise program? If so, has your current problem affected it?

☐ What foods make up your typical daily diet?

☐ Do you take vitamins, calcium, protein, or other food supplements?

☐ What is your current weight? What is it normally?

☐ Have you been constipated?

Related medical history

☐ Have you noticed any other signs or symptoms, such as a fever or a rash?

☐ Have you ever had any injury to a bone, muscle, ligament, cartilage, joint, or tendon? If so, what was the injury? How and when did it occur? How was it treated? Have you experienced any aftereffects?

☐ Have you had any surgery on a bone, muscle, ligament, cartilage, joint, or tendon? When was it done? What was the outcome?

☐ Have you had X-rays of bones in the past? What was the result?

☐ Have you had blood or urine tests because of a muscle or bone problem? What was the result?

☐ Have you ever had fluid removed from a joint or a biopsy performed?

☐ Has anyone in your family had osteoporosis, gout, arthritis, or tuberculosis?

Getting ready for the assessment

Take the equipment needed for a musculoskeletal assessment to the patient's room. Include a measuring tape and marking pen. Wash your hands and explain the procedure to the patient. Ask him to undress (except for his undershorts) before you proceed with the assessment.

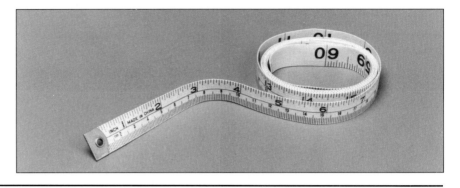

Evaluating posture and mobility

Whenever possible, observe the patient's stance (near right) and movements. For example, notice his gait and general coordination as he walks into his room. If he's already in the room, ask him to walk to the door, turn around, and walk back toward you.

Watch the patient walk (far right). His torso should sway only slightly, his arms should swing naturally at his sides, and his gait should be even. Expect an erect posture.

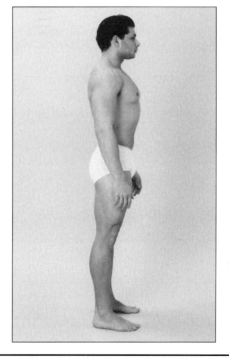
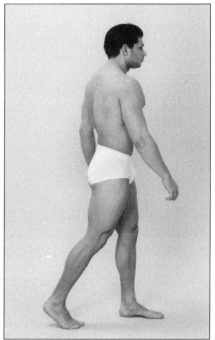

As the patient walks, observe how his foot meets the floor: It should flatten and bear the body's weight completely (near right). As he pushes off with his foot, his toes should flex (far right). Expect the foot in midswing (in the "swing" phase of the gait) to clear the floor and pass the other leg.

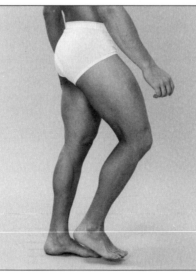
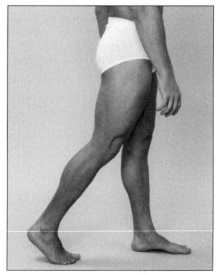

Inspecting the head and neck

Observe lateral motion of the head. Ask the patient to try to touch his right ear to his right shoulder and his left ear to his left shoulder. The usual ROM is 40 degrees on each side.

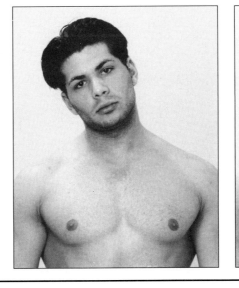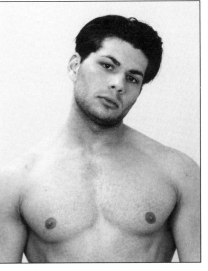

Ask the patient to flex his neck by touching his chin to his chest (near right) and then to extend his neck by pointing his chin toward the ceiling (far right). Normally, the neck flexes forward 45 degrees and extends backward 55 degrees.

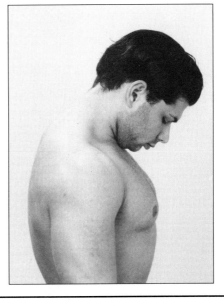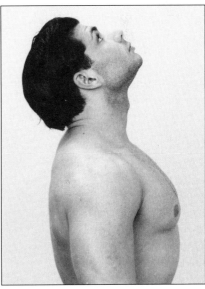

Assess rotation. Ask the patient to turn his head to each side while keeping his trunk still. Normally, the chin will be parallel to the shoulders.

Finally, ask the patient to move his head in a circular motion. Normal rotation is 70 degrees.

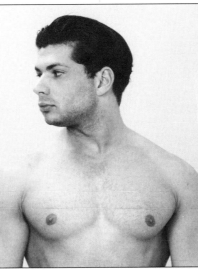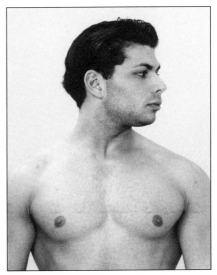

Palpate the neck area for tenderness or crepitation during movement. Stand facing the patient with one hand placed lightly on each side of his neck. Ask him to turn his head from side to side and then flex his neck forward and extend it backward. Feel for any lumps or tender areas as he moves his neck.

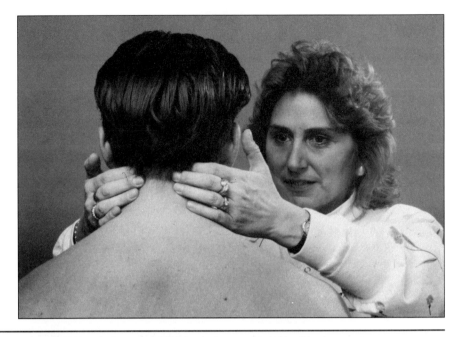

To evaluate the ROM of the jaw area—the temporomandibular joint (TMJ)—place the tips of your first two or three fingers over the TMJ site in front of the middle of the ear (near right). Ask the patient to open and close his mouth. Drop your fingers into the depressed area over the joint (far right), and note the motion of the mandible. Normally, a person can open and close the jaw and protract and retract the mandible easily.

If you hear or palpate a click as the patient's mouth opens, suspect an improperly aligned jaw.

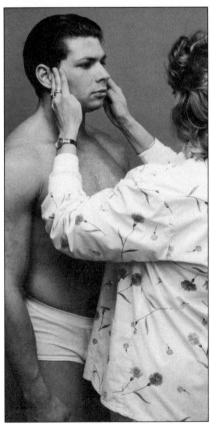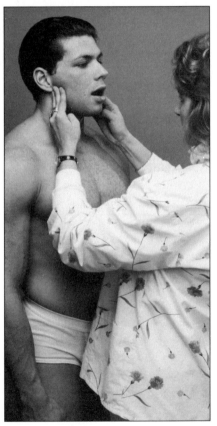

Checking spinal alignment

Next, observe the patient's spine. Have him remove enough clothing for you to assess spinal curvature (from the lateral and the posterior positions). Observe the patient's standing profile. Along the spine, you should see a reverse "S" shape.

If the patient has pronounced lordosis, the lumbar spine will be abnormally concave (inset, near right). If he has pronounced kyphosis, the thoracic curve will be abnormally round (inset, far right).

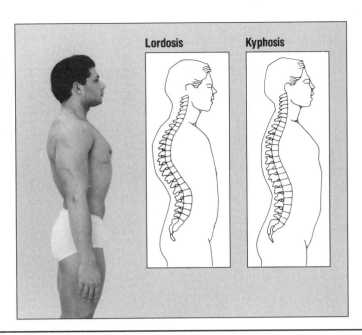

Lordosis   Kyphosis

Next, observe the spine posteriorly. Face the patient's back as he continues to stand. The spine should be in midline position without deviation to either side. Any lateral deviation suggests scoliosis.

To assess for scoliosis, have the patient bend at the waist. This provides a better angle from which to assess a spinal deviation. Normally, the spine remains at midline.

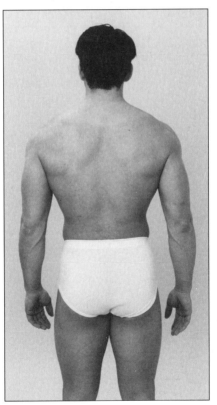

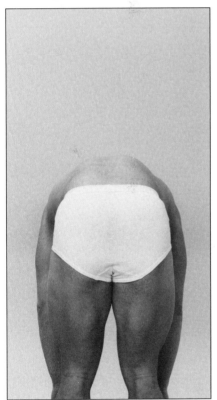

To assess the range of spinal movement, have the patient straighten up. Place the end of the measuring tape at the nape of his neck. Holding the tape in position with one hand, extend it to the patient's waist and measure the distance (near right).

Continue to hold the measuring tape in place at the nape of the patient's neck, and ask him to bend forward at the waist (far right). Allow the measuring tape to move at the waist to accommodate the increased distance as the spine flexes. The length of the spine from neck to waist usually increases by at least 2″ (5 cm) when the person bends forward. If it doesn't, assess further for impaired mobility.

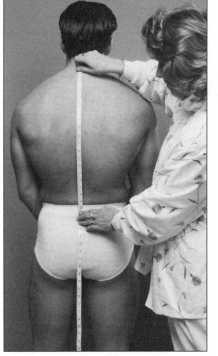
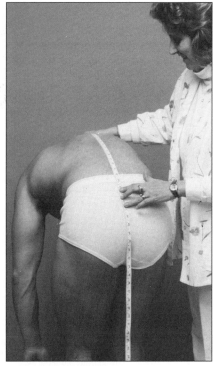

To complete the assessment, palpate the spinal processes and the areas lateral to the spine. Have the patient bend over at the waist with his arms hanging loosely at his sides. Start by palpating the spine with your fingertips. Repeat the palpation using the side of your hand to produce light blows to the areas lateral to the spine. Note any tenderness, swelling, or spasm.

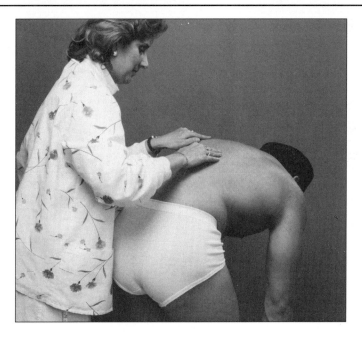

Examining the shoulders and arms

Assess each shoulder for these motions: rotation, flexion, extension, abduction, and adduction.

Start by examining rotation. Ask the patient to straighten his arm and raise it to shoulder level so that it's parallel to the floor. Next, ask him to bend his elbow until his forearm is at a 90-degree angle to his upper arm. Have him extend his fingers and turn his hand palmside down (near right). To assess external rotation, have him bring his forearm up until his fingers point toward the ceiling.

To assess internal rotation, have the patient lower his forearm until his fingers point toward the floor (far right). The normal ROM is 90 degrees in each direction.

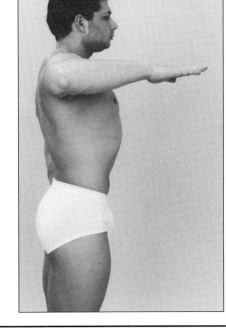
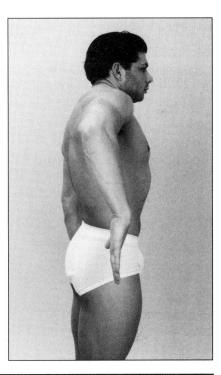

Assess flexion and extension. Have the patient straighten his arm and move it anteriorly from the neutral position at his side to full flexion (180 degrees) with the arm over his head (near right).

To assess extension, have the patient move his arm from the neutral position posteriorly (far right). The normal extension range is 30 to 50 degrees.

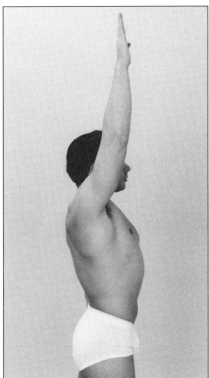
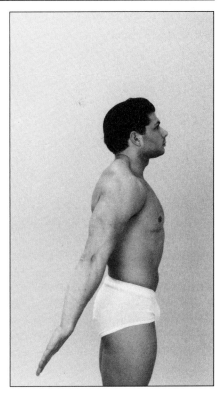

To assess abduction, ask the patient to move his arm laterally from the side of his body (near right). The normal ROM is 180 degrees.

To assess adduction, have the patient move his arm across the front of his body (far right). The normal ROM is 50 degrees.

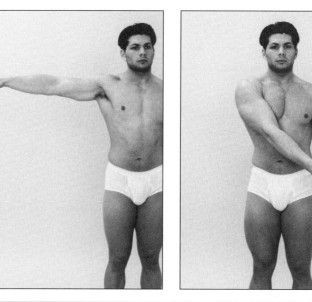

Next, assess the elbow for flexion and extension. Have the patient rest his arm at his side. Ask him to flex his elbow (near right) and then extend his elbow (far right) from this position. The normal ROM is 90 degrees for both flexion and extension.

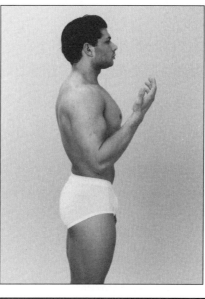
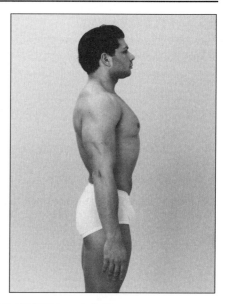

To assess supination and pronation of the elbow, have the patient place the side of his hand on a flat surface with the thumb side up. Ask him to rotate his palm down toward the table for pronation (near right) and upward for supination (far right). The normal angle of elbow rotation is 90 degrees in each direction.

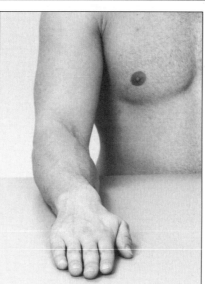
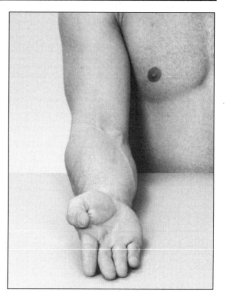

Evaluating the wrists and hands

Ask the patient to rotate his wrist by moving his entire hand—first laterally (near right) and then medially (far right). The expected ROMs are 55 degrees laterally and 20 degrees medially.

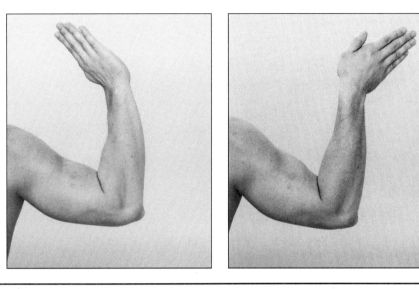

Next, examine the wrist while the patient extends his fingers up toward the ceiling (top) and then down toward the floor (bottom). He should be able to extend his wrist 70 degrees and flex it 90 degrees.

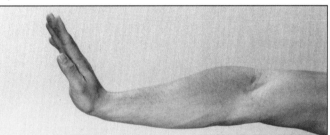

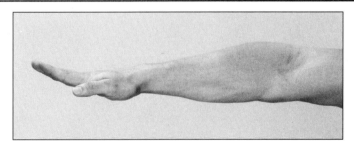

To assess extension and flexion of the metacarpophalangeal joints, ask the patient to keep his wrist still and move only his fingers—first up toward the ceiling (top) and then down toward the floor (bottom). Normal findings are 30 degrees of extension and 90 degrees of flexion.

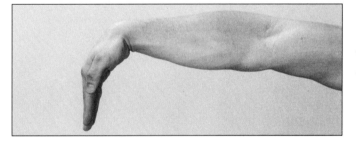

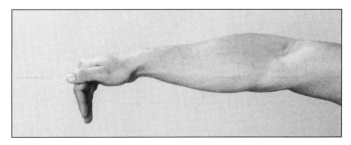

Next, ask the patient to touch his thumb to the little finger of the same hand (near right). He should be able to fold, or flex, his thumb across the palm of his hand so that it touches or points toward the base of the little finger.

To assess flexion of all of the fingers, ask the patient to form a fist (far right).

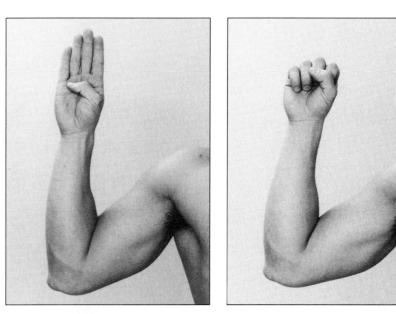

Then have the patient spread his fingers apart to demonstrate abduction (near right) and draw them back together to demonstrate adduction (far right).

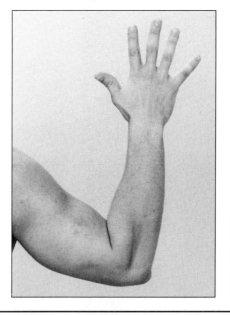
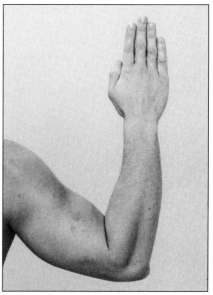

After assessing ROM, use your thumb and index finger to palpate each of the finger joints and the wrist. Note any tenderness, nodules, or bogginess.

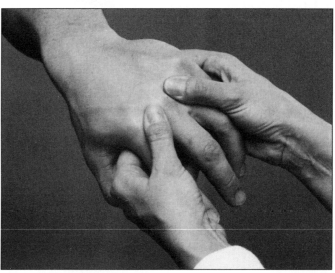

Evaluating the hips and legs

To assess hip flexion, have the patient stand and kick his leg forward. He should be able to kick forward 90 degrees.

▶ *Clinical tip:* If the patient has difficulty standing—because of advanced age, for example—place him in a supine position for this part of the examination.

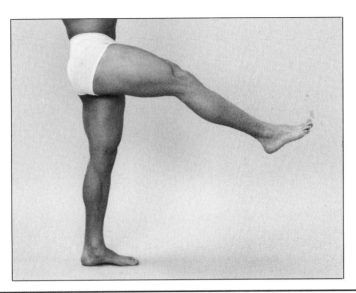

To assess extension, have him kick his leg backward. He should be able to kick backward 35 degrees.

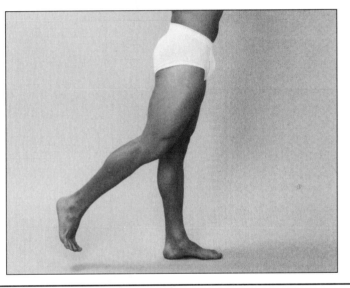

Next, have the patient kick his leg out laterally to assess abduction (near right). The normal ROM for hip abduction is 45 degrees.

Then ask him to swing one leg in front of the other to test adduction (far right). The normal ROM for hip adduction is 30 degrees.

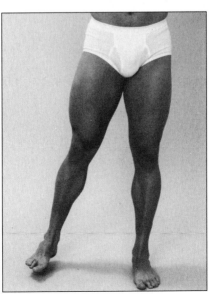
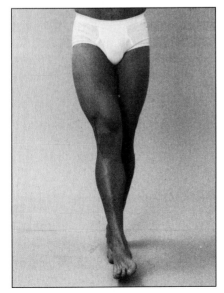

To assess internal rotation of the hip, ask the patient to lift one leg up and, keeping his knee straight, turn his leg and foot medially (near right). Then ask him to turn his leg and foot laterally to assess external rotation (far right). The knee should stay straight during this movement. The normal ROM for internal rotation is 40 degrees; for external rotation, 45 degrees.

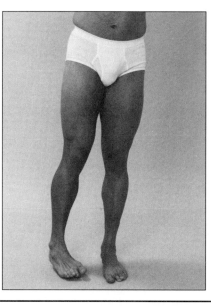
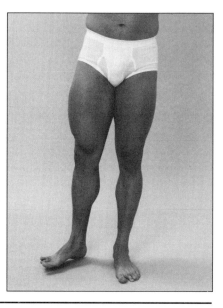

To assess knee flexion if the patient is standing, ask him to bend his knee as if trying to touch his heel to his buttocks (near right). The expected ROM for this maneuver is 130 degrees. If the patient is lying down, have him draw his knee up to his chest. His calf should touch his thigh.

Extension returns the knee to a neutral position of 0 degrees (far right). In some individuals, the knee may be hyperextended 15 degrees normally.

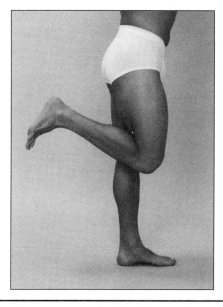
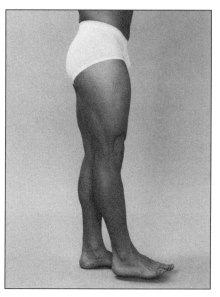

Ask the patient to lie down so that you can palpate the knee. Assess for the "bulge sign," which indicates excess fluid in the joint. Give the medial side of the knee two to four firm strokes to displace any excess fluid (top). Next, tap the lateral aspect of the knee while checking for a fluid wave on the medial aspect (bottom).

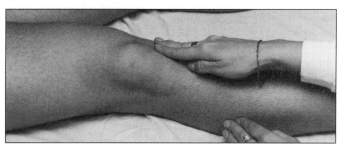
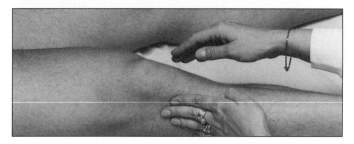

To examine the ankle, have the patient sit in a chair or on the side of the bed. Ask him to show plantar flexion by pointing his toes toward the floor (near right). Then have him demonstrate dorsiflexion by pointing his toes toward his head (far right). The normal ranges are 40 degrees for plantar flexion and 20 degrees for dorsiflexion.

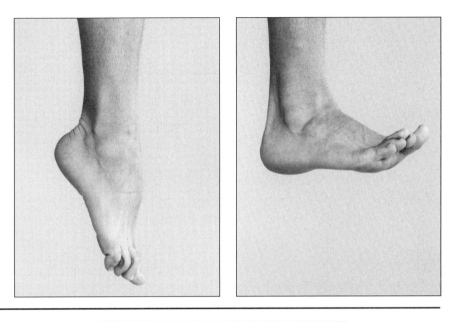

Next, assess ROM. Ask the patient to demonstrate inversion by turning his feet inward (top) and then eversion by turning his feet outward (bottom). Normal ranges are 45 degrees for inversion and 30 degrees for eversion.

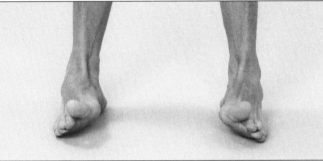

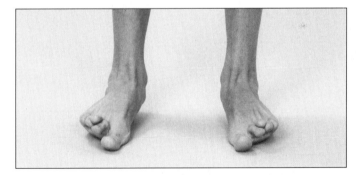

To assess the metatarsophalangeal joints, ask the patient to flex his toes (near right) and then straighten them (far right).

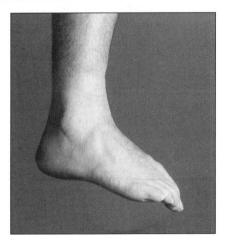

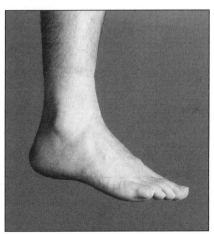

Palpate each toe joint by compressing it with your thumb and your fingers (as shown).

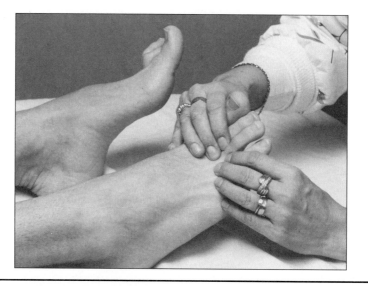

If you suspect that one extremity is longer than the other, measure the length of each limb. Place the ends of the measuring tape at two fixed points. For the leg, use the medial malleolus at the ankle and the anterior iliac spine. The measuring tape should cross over the medial side of the knee.

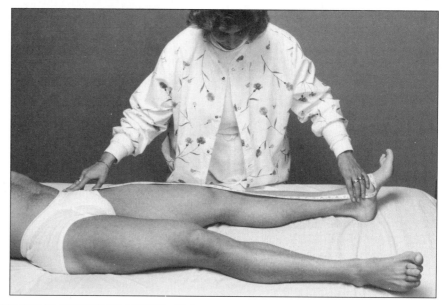

Measure the arm from the acromion process (at the shoulder) to the tip of the middle finger, with the tape draped over the olecranon process (elbow). A difference of no more than ⅜" (1 cm) should exist between the left and right extremities.

Help the patient to a comfortable sitting position. Then wash your hands and document all of your findings.

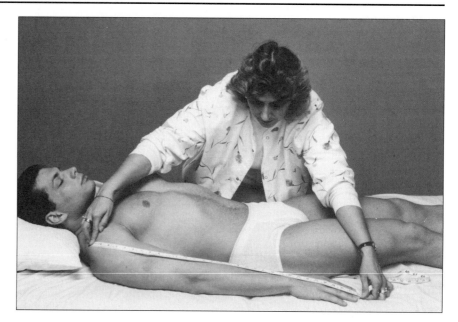

EXAMINING SENSORIMOTOR FUNCTION OF EXTREMITIES

When assessing the sensorimotor function of your patient's extremities, you'll examine movement (including coordination and equilibrium), sensation, and reflexes. In doing so, you may detect signs and symptoms of conditions that may affect your patient's sensorimotor function, such as neurologic infections, diseases, or adverse drug reactions.

CENTRAL NERVOUS SYSTEM

Before assessing sensorimotor function, review nervous system structures and functions as they pertain to the extremities. Remember, the central nervous system (CNS) and the peripheral nervous system are the primary governors of motor and sensory function of the extremities. (See *How the CNS sorts sensorimotor stimuli*, page 164.)

PERIPHERAL NERVOUS SYSTEM

The peripheral nervous system includes the cranial nerves, the spinal nerves, and the autonomic nervous system (see "Examining the Cranial Nerves," pages 60 to 62).

Spinal nerves
Primarily responsible for transmitting impulses between the extremities and the CNS, the spinal nerves come in 31 pairs. Each pair is named for the vertebra immediately below its exit point from the spinal cord. Spinal nerves consist of sensory (afferent) and motor (efferent) neurons.

Spinal sensory neurons transmit stimuli from sensory receptors in the skin, muscle, sensory organs, and viscera to the dorsal horn of the spinal cord. The upper motor neurons of the brain and the lower motor neurons of the cell bodies in the ventral horn carry impulses that affect movement. (See *Neurotransmission and neural pathways*, page 165.)

Reflex actions
The autonomic nervous system can sense and respond to some environmental stimuli without brain involvement. These adaptive responses, called reflexes, occur automatically to protect the body. For example, the eye blinks in response to an approaching object.

Even when the brain can't send a message to a muscle group (because of a spinal cord injury, for example), a stimulus can still elicit reflex activity, provided that the spinal cord is intact at the level of the reflex. The knee-jerk (patellar) reflex exemplifies the activity called a reflex arc. Here's what happens: A sensory receptor detects the stimulus produced by an object striking the patellar tendon and transmits the afferent impulse over an axon, to a spinal nerve, and into the anterior horn of the spinal cord. Here, another sensory neuron connects with a motor neuron via a synapse, and the impulse is transmitted along a branching axon, to a spinal nerve, and to the muscle fibers via the nerve's motor end plate, prompting the muscle to contract and the lower leg to extend with a jerk.

The brain normally suppresses reflex activity. However, if damage to the CNS motor pathways prevents the brain from influencing reflex activity, reflexes become hyperactive.

SPECIAL CONSIDERATIONS

A comprehensive sensorimotor assessment usually takes 1 to 2 hours, depending on the patient's stamina and ability to cooperate. At times, you can perform a sensorimotor screening to evaluate the patient's strength, gait, movement, and sensitivity to touch and pain. However, if the patient exhibits any evidence of motor or sensory dysfunction, you must perform a full assessment.

Before the assessment, talk with the patient to obtain baseline data. (See *Exploring sensorimotor complaints*, page 167.) You'll probably perform motor and sensory assessments simultaneously; however, you may want to categorize your findings (motor, sensory, and reflex assessments, for example) as on the following pages.

Motor function
When assessing motor function of the extremities, you'll evaluate the pyramidal (corticospinal) tract, the extrapyramidal tract, and the cerebellar system. The pyramidal tract mediates voluntary movements

(Text continues on page 166.)

Marie E. Wilson, RN, BSN, CCRN, and *Teresa A. Palmer, RN, MSN, CANP,* contributed to this section. Ms. Wilson is a clinical nurse III at Thomas Jefferson University Hospital, Philadelphia. Ms. Palmer is an assistant clinical professor at the University of Medicine and Dentistry of New Jersey in Newark. The publisher thanks *Doylestown (Pa.) Hospital* and *Hill-Rom,* Batesville, Ind., for their help.

How the CNS sorts sensorimotor stimuli

The central nervous system (CNS), which consists of the brain and spinal cord, processes and interprets voluntary and involuntary motor and sensory signals and controls the peripheral (voluntary) and autonomic (involuntary) nervous systems.

Brain

As the highest-functioning center of the CNS, the brain integrates and interprets all stimuli. Its three distinct regions—the cerebrum, the cerebellum, and the brain stem—initiate and monitor voluntary and involuntary motor activity.

• The cerebrum governs both motor and sensory activity—motor activities from the frontal lobe, sensory activities from the parietal lobe, hearing and smell from the temporal lobe, and vision from the occipital lobe. The lobes of the right cerebral hemisphere control activities on the body's left side; the lobes of the left cerebral hemisphere control activities on the body's right side.

The diencephalon, a division of the cerebrum, contains thalamic structures, notably the thalamus and the hypothalamus. The thalamus relays sensory impulses; the hypothalamus regulates temperature, pituitary hormone production, and water balance.

• The cerebellum contains the major motor and sensory pathways, which facilitate coordinated muscle movements and maintain equilibrium.

• The brain stem, consisting of the midbrain, pons, and medulla oblongata, conducts motor and sensory information to and from the cerebrum to regulate such functions as respiration, hearing, vision, swallowing, and coughing.

Spinal cord

An extension of the brain stem, the spinal cord extends to the lower border of the first lumbar vertebra. It consists of an H-shaped mass of tissue known as gray matter and a mass of encircling white matter encased in and protected by the spinal vertebrae.

Divided into dorsal (posterior) and ventral (anterior) horns, the gray matter relays sensory (afferent) impulses via the dorsal horns and motor (efferent) impulses via the ventral horns. White matter (myelinated axons of sensory and motor nerves) surrounds these horns and forms the ascending and descending tracts of the spinal cord.

Besides transmitting impulses between the peripheral areas of the body and the brain, the spinal cord mediates the reflex arc—the path followed by a nerve impulse in reflex responses.

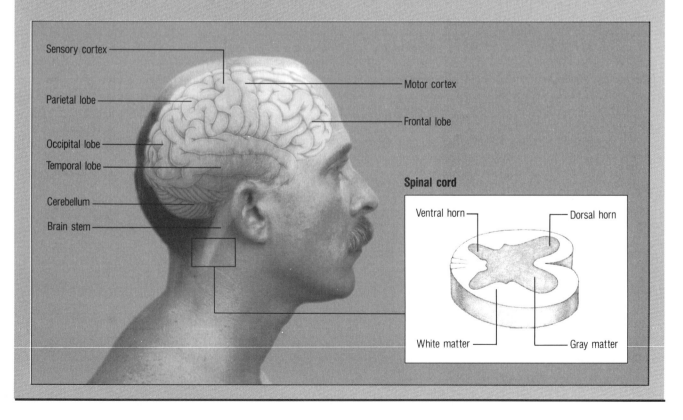

Sensory cortex
Parietal lobe
Occipital lobe
Temporal lobe
Cerebellum
Brain stem
Motor cortex
Frontal lobe

Spinal cord

Ventral horn
Dorsal horn
White matter
Gray matter

Neurotransmission and neural pathways

Neurotransmission—the conduction of impulses in the nervous system—operates through the actions of neurons, specialized cells that detect and transmit stimuli as electrochemical messages or impulses over sensory or motor pathways.

The stimuli that the neurons transmit can be mechanical (touch or pressure), thermal (heat or cold), or chemical (either external chemicals or internal ones such as histamine, a substance released by the body).

Sensory pathways

From sensory receptors located in the skin, muscles, sensory organs, and viscera, sensory impulses travel by afferent, or ascending, pathways to the sensory cortex in the parietal lobe of the brain, where they are then interpreted. Pain and temperature sensations enter the spinal cord through the dorsal horn and immediately cross over to the opposite side of the cord. They then travel to the thalamus via the spinothalamic tract.

Sensations of touch, pressure, and vibration enter the spinal cord via the dorsal root ganglia. These stimuli travel up the cord in the dorsal column to the medulla oblongata, where they cross over to the opposite side and enter the thalamus. The thalamus relays all incoming sensory impulses—except the olfactory ones—to the sensory cortex in the parietal lobe for interpretation.

Motor pathways

Motor (efferent or descending) pathways transmit impulses from the brain to the muscles in the following manner: Motor impulses that originate in the motor cortex of the frontal lobe reach the lower motor neurons of the peripheral nervous system via upper motor neurons of the pyramidal or extrapyramidal tract.

In the pyramidal tract, impulses travel from the motor cortex, through the internal capsule, to the medulla, where they cross over to the opposite side and continue down the spinal cord. In the anterior horn of the spinal cord, impulses are relayed to the lower motor neurons, which carry them along the spinal cord and peripheral nerves to the muscles, producing a motor response.

Motor impulses that regulate involuntary muscle tone and muscle control travel along the extrapyramidal tract from the premotor area of the frontal lobe to the pons of the brain stem, where they cross over to the opposite side. The impulses then travel down the spinal cord to the ventral horn, where they are relayed to the lower motor neurons, which carry the impulses to the muscles.

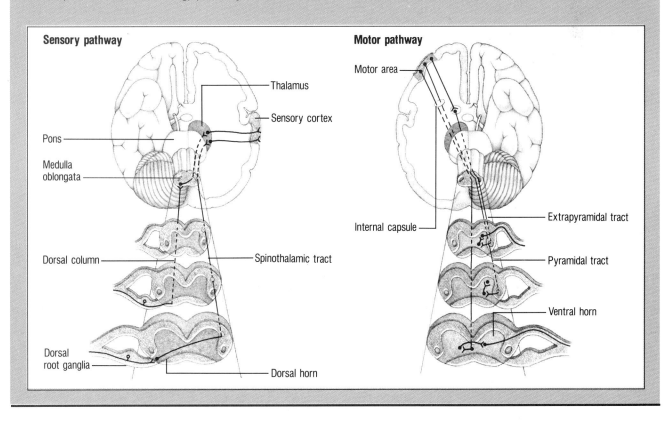

Sensory pathway
- Thalamus
- Sensory cortex
- Pons
- Medulla oblongata
- Dorsal column
- Spinothalamic tract
- Dorsal root ganglia
- Dorsal horn

Motor pathway
- Motor area
- Internal capsule
- Extrapyramidal tract
- Pyramidal tract
- Ventral horn

Identifying dermatomes

The body surface is sectioned into areas called dermatomes. The skin area within each dermatome is enervated with sensory (afferent) nerve fibers from an individual spinal root, which determines the identity of each dermatome. For example, cervical (C) spinal nerves enervate 8 dermatomes, thoracic (T) spinal nerves enervate 12 dermatomes, lumbar (L) spinal nerves enervate 5 dermatomes, and sacral (S) spinal nerves enervate 5 dermatomes.

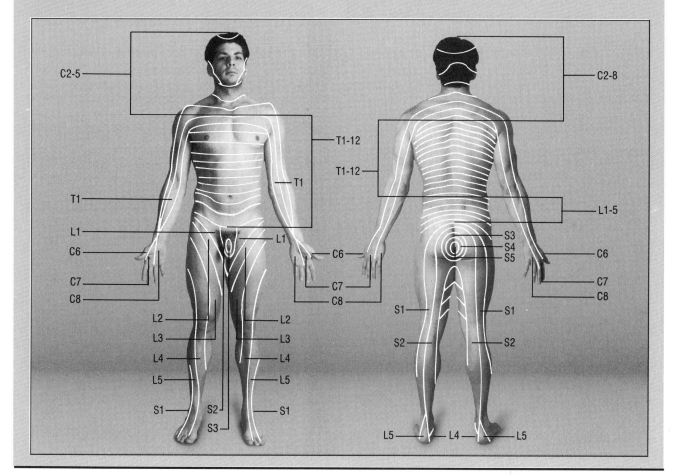

originating in the brain's motor cortex as well as complex and delicate movements. The extrapyramidal tract governs muscle tone and controls gross body movements such as walking. The cerebellar system coordinates muscle activity and maintains equilibrium and posture.

During this part of the assessment, evaluate the patient's muscle size, tone, and strength as well as his movement. Although testing all muscle groups is impractical, examining a few major ones provides an overall impression of the patient's muscle status. To assess muscle strength, have the patient perform active range-of-motion (ROM) exercises against your resistance. Use a standard muscle-strength scale to record your findings.

A word of caution: To ensure that the patient can be examined safely, assess his level of consciousness and stamina before beginning. If he exhibits syncope or serious fatigue, defer the balance and coordination portion of the assessment until his condition improves.

Sensory function

In this part of the assessment, you'll test the patient's perception of light touch, pain, temperature, and vibration. You'll also test his proprioception (position sense) and discriminative sense. Note areas with no sensation (anesthesia), diminished sensation (hypoesthesia), or heightened sensation (hyperesthesia). Use a dermatome chart to mark areas with abnormal sensation. (See *Identifying dermatomes*.)

ASSESSMENT CHECKLIST

Exploring sensorimotor complaints

Before you assess sensorimotor function in your patient's extremities, obtain pertinent baseline data. First ask the patient about his chief complaint. Then focus your questions on neuromotor and neurosensory function. Use the following questions as a guide:

☐ What prompted you to seek treatment?
☐ Would you rate your muscle strength as superior, good, average, below average, or poor? Why?
☐ Have you noticed a change in muscle strength? If so, when did you first notice it?
☐ Do you have paralysis or weakness in any part of your body? If so, where? When did you first notice it? Describe the symptoms.
☐ Have you ever had tremors, spasms, or shakiness in your muscles? If so, how often does the condition occur? Have you been treated for it by a doctor?

☐ Do you ever experience problems with your gait or balance?
☐ Do you ever fall because you lose your balance?
☐ Would you rate your coordination as superior, good, average, below average, or poor? Why?
☐ Do you drop things periodically? If so, are you doing it more often? Provide details.
☐ Have you noticed any changes in your ability to feel textures, temperatures, or other sensations?
☐ Have you ever burned yourself without realizing it? Provide details.
☐ Have you ever had a stroke? If so, give details.
☐ Have you ever been treated by a neurologist or a neurosurgeon? If so, for what? Is he still treating you? Can you describe the treatment?
☐ Do you take any medications (for example, aspirin or anticoagulants)?

When testing touch, pain, and temperature sensations, compare the distal and proximal areas of each extremity, and scatter the stimulus pattern so that the patient can't respond to an anticipated stimulus. Start with the shoulders, move down the arms, testing the inner and outer aspects of each forearm, and then test the hands and fingers. When testing the lower extremities, start with the anterior thighs, move down to the medial and lateral aspects of the calves, and then test the toes. Be sure to change the pace of the testing to ensure that the patient isn't just responding to a repetitive rhythm.

Reflex function

Evaluating your patient's reflexes involves testing both deep tendon and superficial reflexes. For best results, explain the tests to the patient, assure him that they aren't painful, and help him to relax.

In deep tendon reflex tests, the limb should be relaxed and the joint in midposition (a knee or elbow should be flexed at a 45-degree angle, for ex-

ample). Because the cerebral cortex may dull the patient's response if he focuses on his performance, distract him by asking him to focus on an object across the room.

Always test deep tendon reflexes from head to toe. And remember to test and compare each reflex contralaterally, keeping in mind that the patient's dominant side is usually stronger than his nondominant side. Determine whether your patient is right- or left-handed, and keep this difference in mind when making comparisons.

To elicit a deep tendon reflex, tap the tendon lightly but firmly with a reflex hammer. Grade the response on a scale of 0 to 4.

When testing superficial reflexes, you'll stimulate the patient's skin or mucous membranes by poking and prodding or administering hot or cold stimuli. To document your findings, use a plus sign (+) to indicate an active reflex and a minus sign (−) to indicate an absent reflex.

Getting ready for the examination

Assemble the equipment you'll need at the patient's bedside. To assess motor function, obtain a tape measure and a sheet or bath blanket to cover the patient when you test ROM.

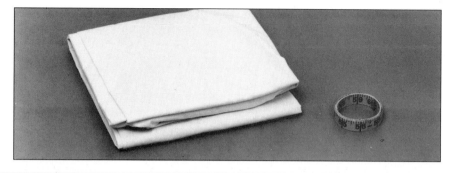

To assess sensory function, gather a safety pin, a tuning fork, a pencil, several cotton balls, two paper clips, two test tubes, and a few common objects, such as a spoon, a cup, and a key.

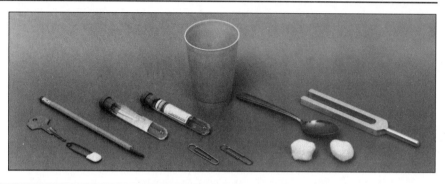

To assess the patient's reflexes, obtain a reflex hammer and a tongue blade.

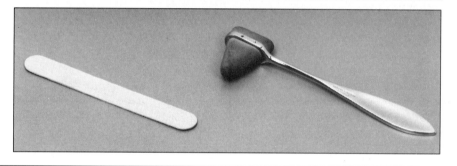

Evaluating motor function

Wash your hands and provide privacy for the patient. Explain the procedure, and inform her that she'll perform various movements during the examination. Reassure her that these movements won't cause discomfort or embarrassment. Then assist her into an upright sitting or a semi-Fowler position.

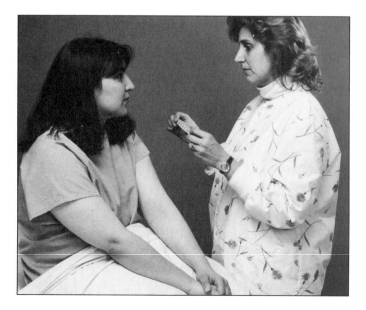

Checking muscle size

Inspect the muscle groups of the arms and legs. Begin by holding the patient's arm and observing the symmetry of the large muscles. Note any atrophy or abnormal muscle movements, such as tics, tremors, or fasciculations. Repeat the inspection on the patient's other arm.

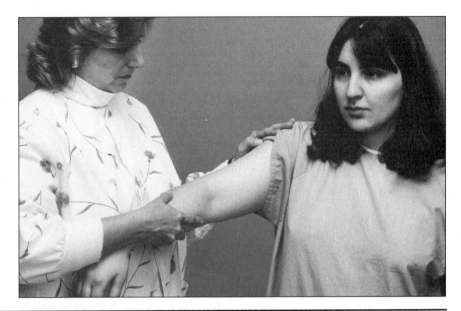

Measure the circumference of the patient's upper arms. Always measure at the widest point of the muscle group. Compare the measurements for each arm and note any differences.

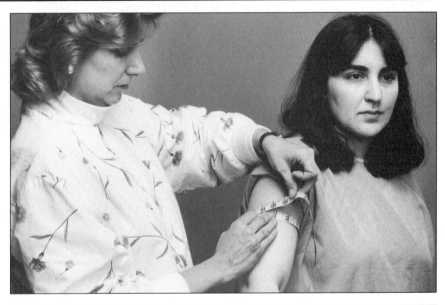

Have the patient lie on her back with her legs relaxed and slightly flexed. Measure the circumference of the right and left thighs at the widest part.

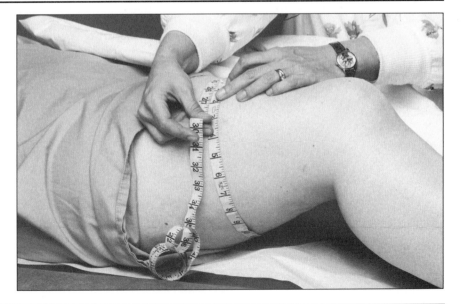

With the patient's legs still in the relaxed, flexed position, measure the circumference of her calf muscles. Compare your findings for each calf and note any differences.

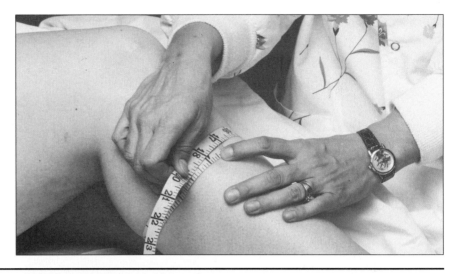

Testing muscle tone

To evaluate muscle tone (muscle resistance to passive stretching) in the patient's arms, have her sit or stand. Support her elbow with one hand, grasp her wrist with your other hand, and move her arm through passive ROM exercises. Repeat this test on the other arm.

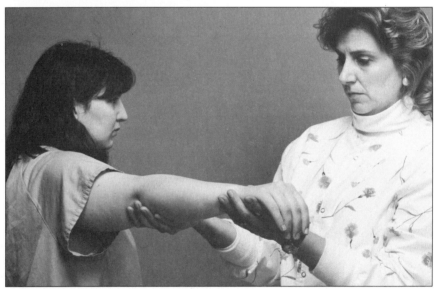

When you finish, let the patient's arm drop to her side. It should fall easily. A rigid arm suggests heightened muscle tone, possibly from an upper motor neuron lesion. A flaccid arm suggests diminished muscle tone, possibly from a lower motor neuron lesion.

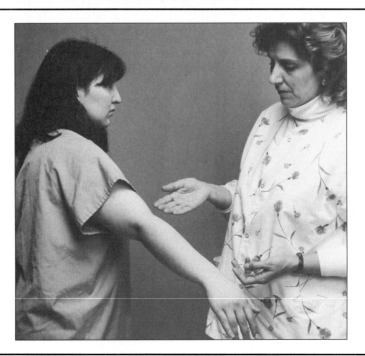

Continue by testing leg muscle tone. Have the patient lie on her back. As you did with the arm, guide the hip through passive ROM exercises. Support the patient's knee with one hand, position your other hand under her heel, and guide the leg through its complete ROM. Repeat the exercise on the opposite leg.

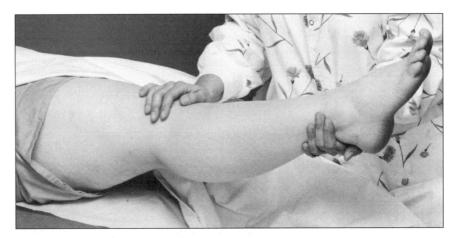

After completing ROM exercises, hold the patient's leg about 12″ to 15″ (30 to 38 cm) above the mattress or examination table, and let the leg drop. Note the position of the leg after it falls. An externally rotated position is an abnormal finding.

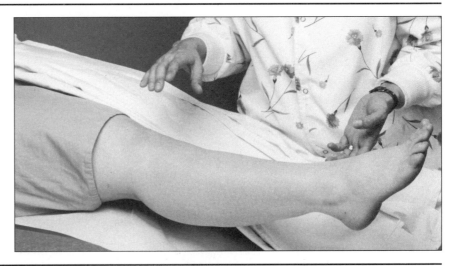

Evaluating muscle strength

Grade muscle strength on a scale of 1 to 5, as follows:

5/5: normal (patient moves joint through full ROM and against gravity with full resistance)

4/5: good (patient completes ROM against gravity with moderate resistance)

3/5: fair (patient completes ROM against gravity only)

2/5: poor (patient completes ROM with gravity eliminated)

1/5: trace (patient's attempt at muscle contraction is palpable, but without joint movement)

0/5: zero (no evidence of muscle contraction).

Test muscle strength with the patient sitting or standing. Begin with the shoulders and the trapezius muscles. Have her shrug her shoulders, and observe for equal height and movement on both sides.

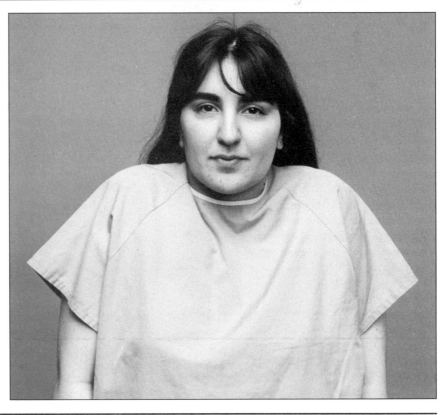

Next, place your hands on the patient's shoulders and have her shrug her shoulders against your resistance.

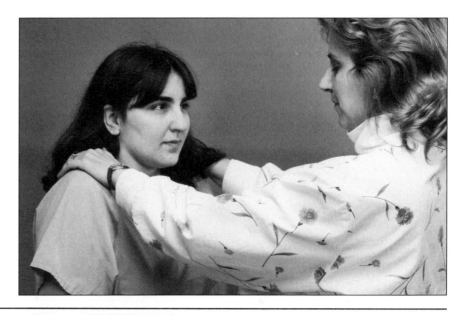

Now test shoulder girdle strength. Instruct the patient to extend her arms in front of her, palms down, and hold the position for 30 seconds.

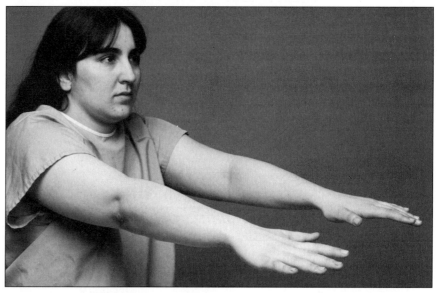

If the patient can hold her arms outstretched, further test her strength by placing your hands on her forearms and pressing downward as she resists. Record your impression of the patient's ability to resist both gravity (holding her arms out) and force (resisting your pressure on her forearms).

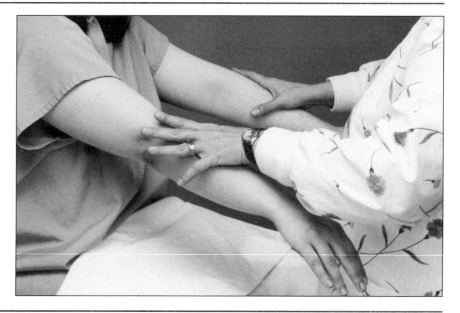

Next, assess the deltoid muscles by testing the patient's ability to abduct her arms. Have her hold her arm at her side. Then place one hand over the deltoid muscle. Support her straightened arm at the elbow with your other hand.

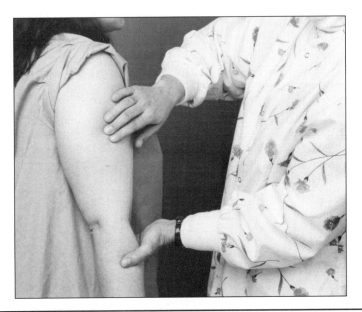

Ask her to abduct her arm to a horizontal position and, as she does so, palpate for a contraction of the deltoid muscle. Repeat this exercise with the other arm.

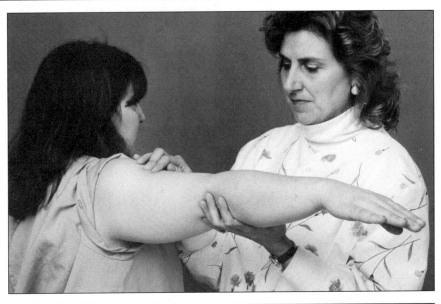

If the patient can perform this movement, repeat the procedure while applying resistance. Be sure to check the contralateral muscle group.

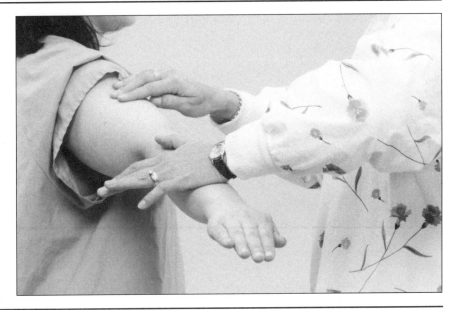

Next, assess the strength and movement of the biceps muscles. Ask the patient to hold her lower arm at a 90-degree angle to her upper arm. Put one of your hands on the biceps muscle, and grasp her wrist with your other hand.

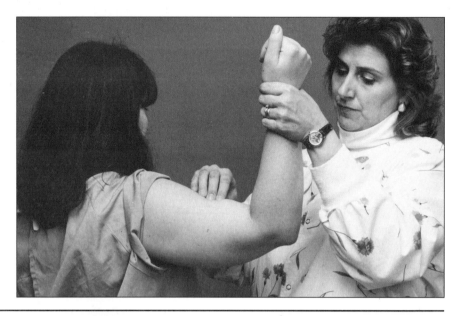

Have the patient flex her forearm against your resistance. Palpate for contraction of the biceps muscle.

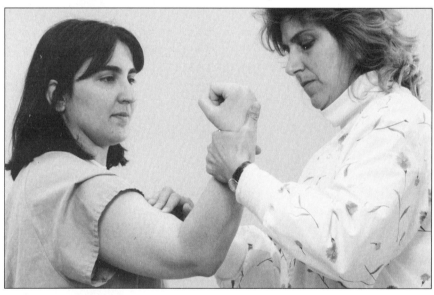

To test triceps muscle function, have the patient extend her elbow by holding her lower arm at a 90-degree angle to her upper arm. Place one of your hands on the triceps muscle, and grasp her wrist with your other hand.

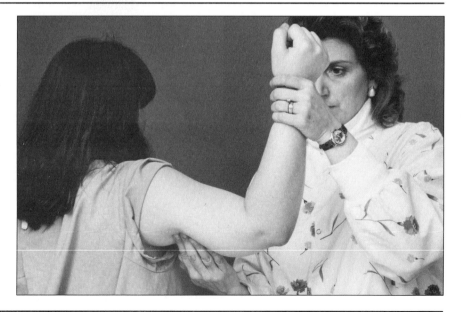

Have the patient extend her forearm against your resistance. Palpate for contraction of the triceps muscle.

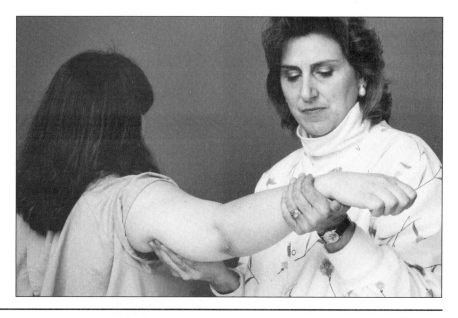

To test the strength and motion of the extensor carpi radialis, have the patient bend her wrist back toward her shoulder (dorsiflexion).

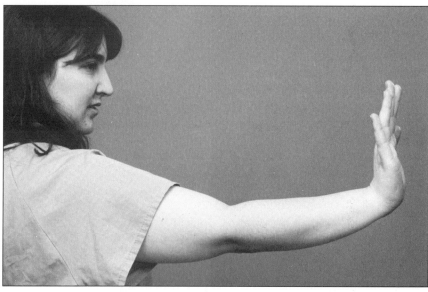

Then place your hand on the back of her hand, and ask her to maintain her position against your resistance. You may place your other hand under the patient's lower arm to support it.

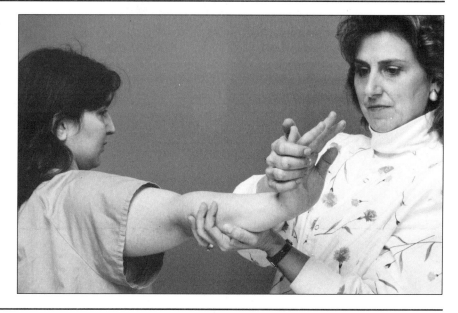

To test wrist extension, ask the patient to dorsiflex her wrist. Place the palm of your hand against the palm of her hand, and support her lower arm with your other hand. Ask her to straighten her wrist against your resistance.

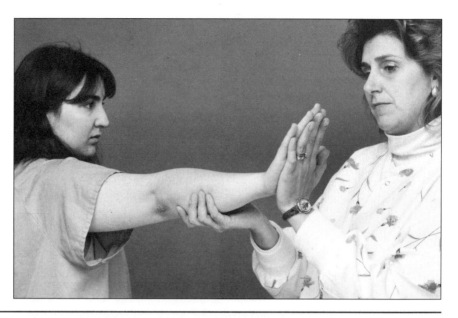

To assess hand muscle strength, do the hand grip test. Have the patient grasp your index and middle fingers firmly.

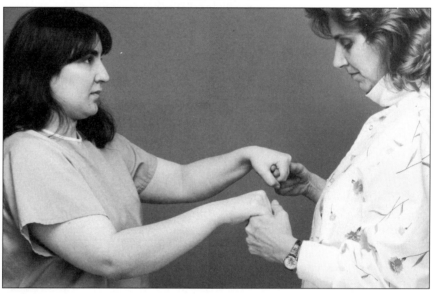

To test hip (iliopsoas) muscle strength, have the patient lie down. Instruct her to raise her knee while you support her leg. Place one hand under the ankle and the other hand above her knee on the anterior thigh. Ask her to keep flexing her hip against your resistance.

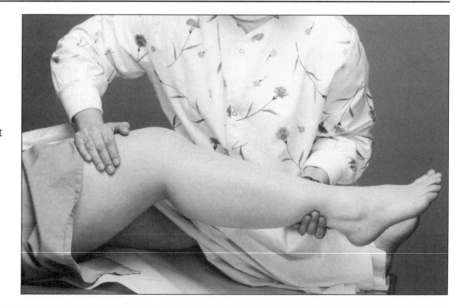

To assess strength in the quadriceps muscle, have the patient extend her knee. Support her lower leg with one hand while she bends her knee slightly. Then place your other hand at the midpoint of the anterior thigh, and ask her to try to straighten her leg against your resistance. Palpate the contraction of the quadriceps muscle.

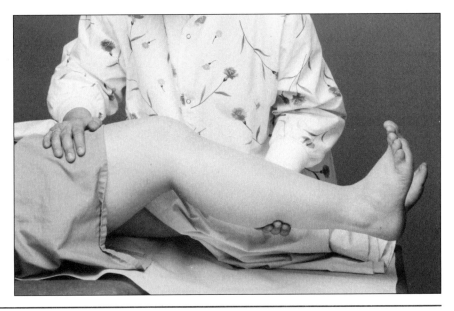

To assess the ankle (anterior tibialis) muscle, have the patient extend and relax her leg. Place your hand on the dorsal surface of her foot, and ask her to dorsiflex her ankle against your resistance.

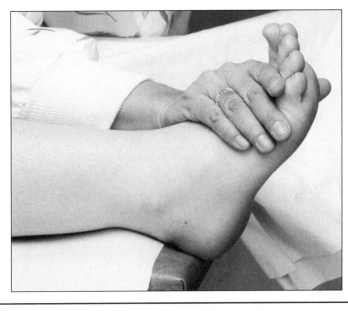

To evaluate the calf (gastrocnemius) muscle, assess plantar flexion in the ankle. Position the patient on her side. Place one hand on her calf and the other hand on the plantar surface of her foot. Ask her to press her foot against your resistance. Palpate the contraction of the calf muscle.

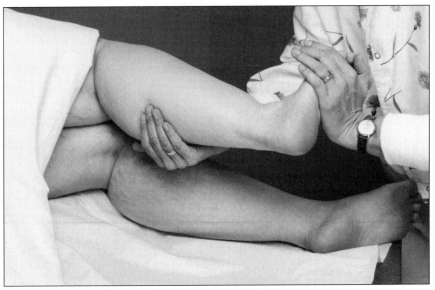

Evaluating balance and coordination

To assess cerebellar function, evaluate coordination of the patient's whole body as well as of her extremities. Begin this part of the physical examination by observing her general balance and coordination. Can she sit upright without support? Can she sit on the side of the bed or examination table? Can she stand? Remember, her ability to sit or stand may be diminished by weakness unrelated to cerebellar dysfunction.

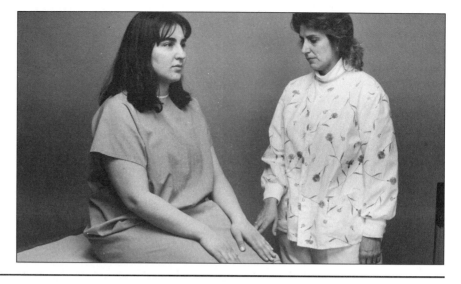

Observe the patient as she walks across the room, turns, and walks back. Note any imbalances or abnormalities in her gait.

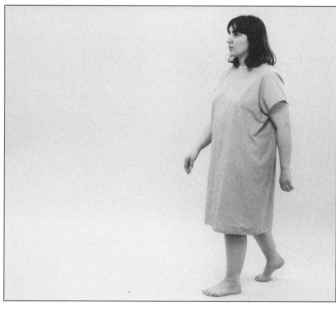

Next, ask the patient to walk heel-to-toe (with one foot directly in front of the other) and observe her balance. Stand nearby to reassure her and to provide assistance if she becomes unsteady. Don't ask her to walk heel-to-toe or perform the Romberg test if she has any weakness or gait abnormalities.

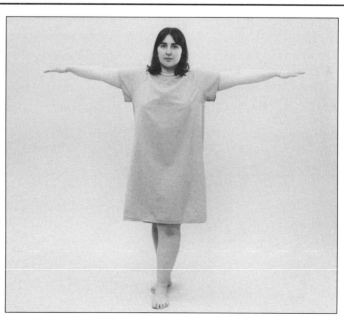

To perform the Romberg test, ask the patient to stand with her feet together, her eyes open, and her arms at her sides. Stand nearby, with your arms outstretched on either side of the patient so that you can support her if she sways (near right). Observe her balance.

Then have the patient close her eyes (far right). Note whether she loses her balance or sways.

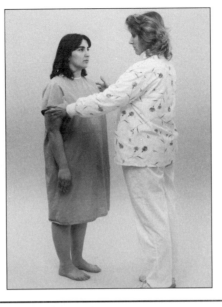 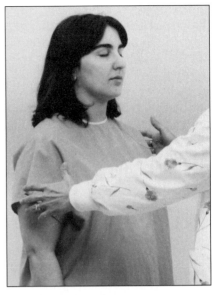

To evaluate coordination of the patient's extremities, test point-to-point movements as well as rapid skilled and rapid alternating movements. To test point-to-point coordination, stand about 2' (0.6 m) away from the patient. Hold up your index finger; then ask the patient to close her eyes and to touch the tip of her index finger to yours.

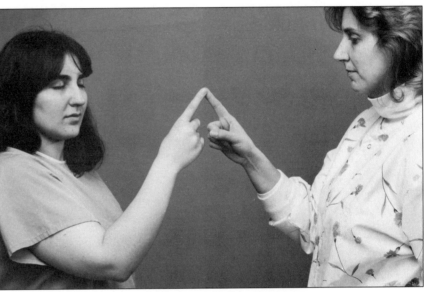

Next, with her eyes still closed, have the patient move her finger from your finger to her nose. Ask her to repeat this exercise several times, gradually increasing her speed. Then have her perform the test using her other index finger.

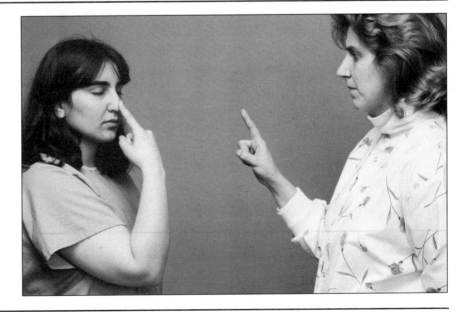

To test rapid skilled movement, ask the patient to touch the thumb of her hand to her index finger (near right) and then to each of her remaining fingers (far right). Instruct her to increase her speed as she repeats each series of movements. Observe for smoothness and accuracy. Repeat the test on her other hand.

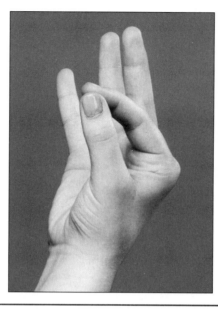 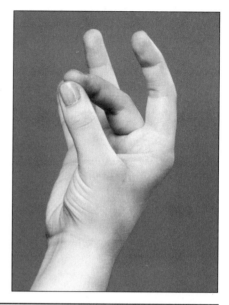

Next, have the patient lie down. Instruct her to touch the heel of her left foot to the shin of her right leg (near right) and run her heel down the shin (far right) to her ankle. Have her repeat this exercise with her right foot.

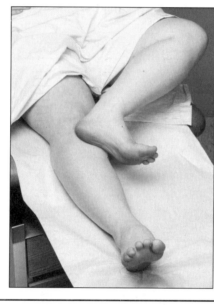 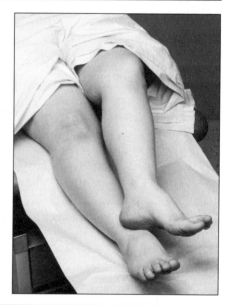

To assess rapid alternating movement, have the patient sit with her palms face down on her thighs (near right). Instruct her to turn her palms up (far right) and then down, gradually increasing her speed with each repetition.

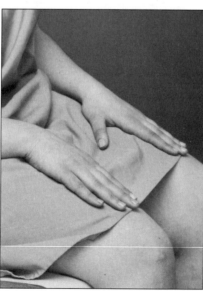 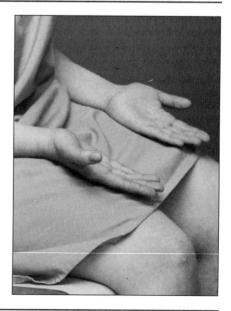

Evaluating sensory function

Inform the patient that she'll need to keep her eyes closed throughout most of this assessment. Begin by testing her response to light touch. Direct her to close her eyes and extend her right arm in front of her. Ask her to tell you when she feels something and what she feels. Then lightly touch her forearm with a cotton ball.

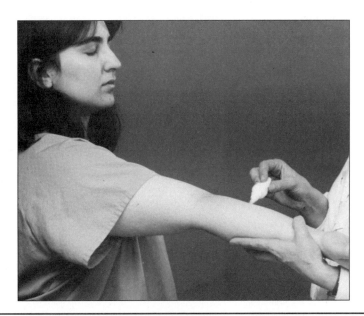

Testing pain

Have the patient keep her eyes closed and extend her arm. Using a safety pin (or a similar sharp object), lightly touch her forearm with the sharp end (near right) and then the blunt end (far right). Be careful not to pierce the skin with the pin's point.

Ask the patient to identify each sensation as sharp or dull. Test both arms, the trunk, and both legs. Discard the testing implement in a biohazard container.

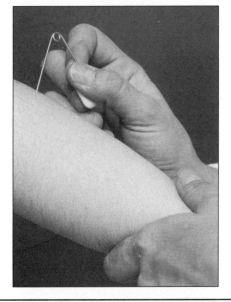
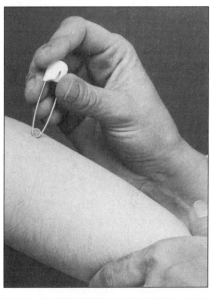

Testing temperature

To test temperature sensation, prepare two test tubes or containers, one with hot—but not too hot—water (about 105° F [40.5° C]) and the other with cold water. Ask the patient to close her eyes. Touch the hot test tube to her cheek for about 1 second. Next, touch the cold test tube to her cheek. Ask the patient to describe the temperature she feels and where she feels it. Continue the test on the opposite cheek and on both arms and legs.

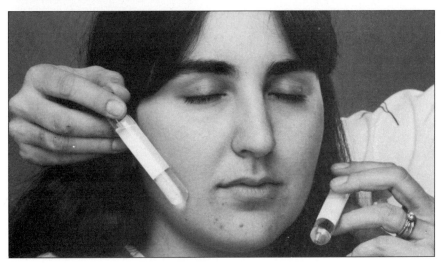

Testing vibrations

To test vibratory sensation, ask the patient to close her eyes. Strike a tuning fork against the heel of your hand to begin the vibrations.

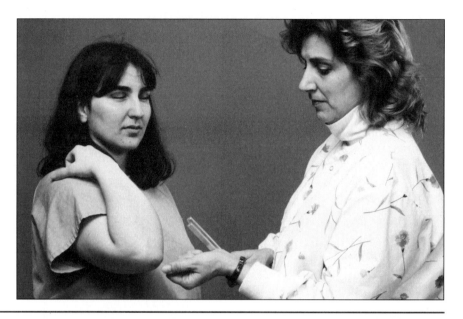

Holding the instrument by the stem, place the end of the tuning fork against the patient's elbow. After a few seconds, touch the top of the tuning fork to stop the vibrations.

Ask the patient to tell you when she feels the vibrations and when she feels them stop. Repeat the procedure on the patient's opposite elbow and on her knees, ankles, and great toes. Also perform this test over any bony area, such as the sternum, the ribs, and the clavicles. If you find an area of diminished sensitivity, repeat the test several times to confirm your findings.

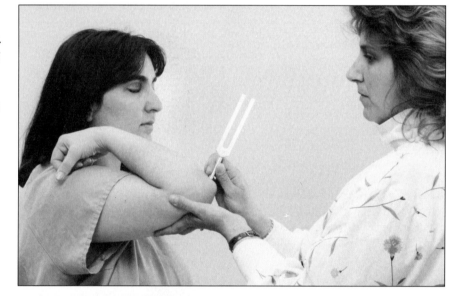

Testing proprioception

To test the patient's proprioception, hold her index finger between your thumb and index finger. Ask her to close her eyes while you move her finger up and down. After each movement, ask the patient to tell you in which direction you moved her finger. Repeat this test on the wrists, ankles, and toes.

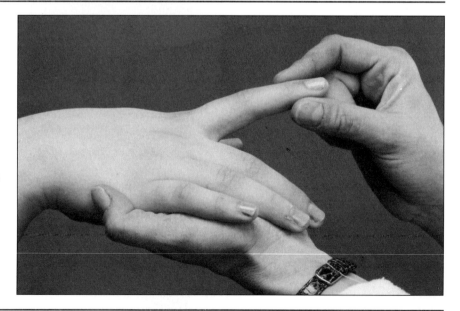

Testing discrimination

To test the patient's discriminative sense, start with common objects, such as a spoon, a paper clip, a cup, and a key.

Ask the patient to close her eyes while you place an object in her hand. Then ask her to identify the object as she fingers it with eyes closed. The ability to identify an object from its size and shape is called stereognosis.

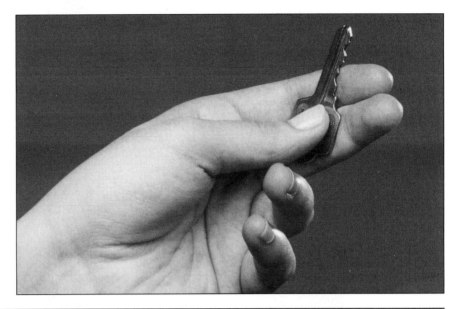

Next, have the patient close her eyes and open her hand palm up. Use your finger or a blunt pencil to draw a large number on her palm. Ask her to identify the number you drew.

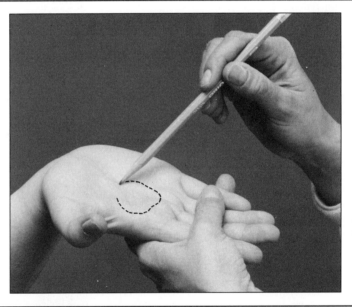

To test two-point discrimination, open the ends of two paper clips. Ask the patient to close her eyes while you touch a finger pad in two places simultaneously with the ends of each paper clip (near right). Alternate this touch using the end of only one paper clip (far right).

Ask the patient to distinguish between one- and two-point touches. As you repeat this test, bring the two points closer together. A patient can usually discriminate between one point and two points if the two points are at least 5 mm apart on the finger pads.

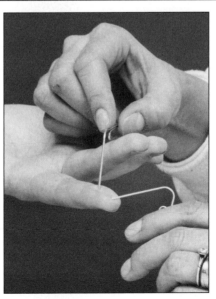
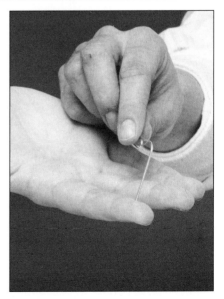

Next, test point localization. Ask the patient to close her eyes while you briefly touch her skin with the end of the paper clip (near right). Then ask her to open her eyes and point to the spot you touched (far right). Repeat this test randomly over the patient's body.

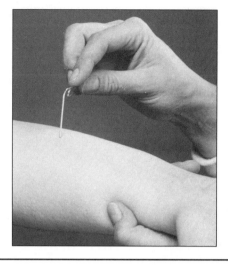
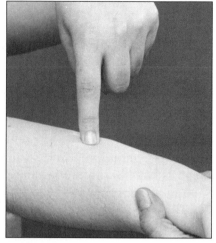

Now touch two cotton balls simultaneously to the patient's right and left sides while the patient keeps her eyes closed. Ask her to identify where she feels the cotton balls. Normally, the patient will feel the stimuli on both sides.

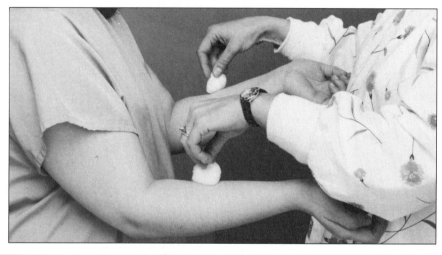

Evaluating reflexes

You'll evaluate the intensity of the patient's reflexes in the following sequence: deep tendon reflexes (such as the biceps reflex), superficial reflexes (such as the plantar reflex), and primitive reflexes (such as the grasp and snout reflexes). Grade reflex intensity on a scale of 0 to 4, as follows:

0: absent
1+: present but diminished
2+: normal
3+: increased
4+: hyperactive, clonic.

Record the patient's reflex scores and their exact locations. If helpful, draw a stick figure, and write the scores at the proper locations on the figure. (Color areas in photo indicate locations of some reflexes.)

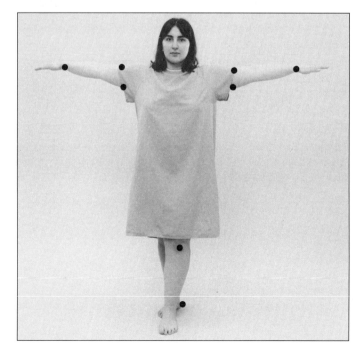

Testing deep tendon reflexes

Assess the patient's biceps reflex by flexing her elbow slightly and holding it with your thumb pressing tightly against the biceps muscle. Then grasp the reflex hammer and strike it against your thumb.

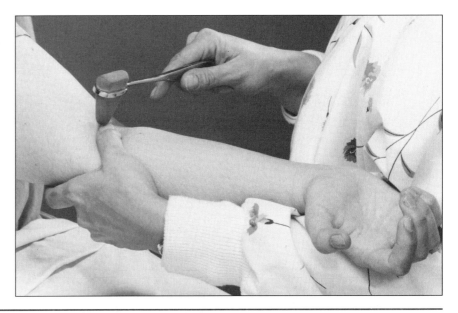

The patient's biceps muscle should contract, causing the arm to flex slightly at the elbow.

As with all sensorimotor tests, repeat this test on the patient's opposite side.

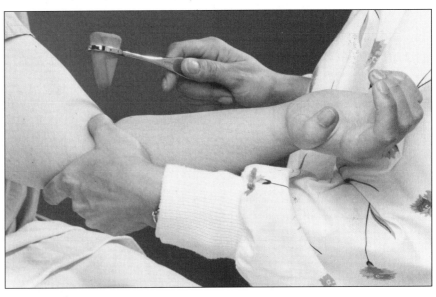

Test the patient's triceps reflex by flexing her arm at the elbow and holding it at the wrist with one hand. With your other hand, grasp the reflex hammer and strike the tendon of the triceps muscle directly over the patient's elbow.

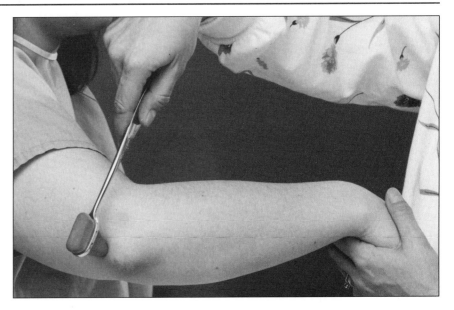

The muscle should contract, causing the patient to extend her arm at the elbow.

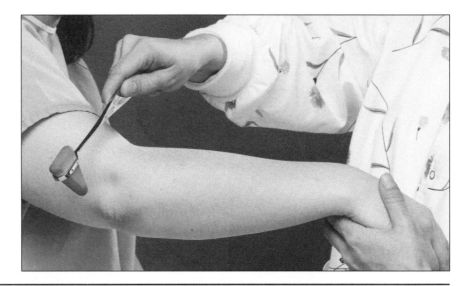

To test the brachioradialis reflex, hold the patient's hand slightly below the wrist, with her palm down. Grasping the reflex hammer, strike the tendon of the patient's brachioradialis muscle, normally located 1″ to 2″ (2.5 to 5 cm) above the wrist (near right).

The patient's forearm should rotate laterally, causing her palm to turn upward (far right).

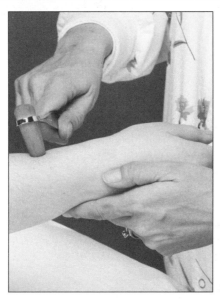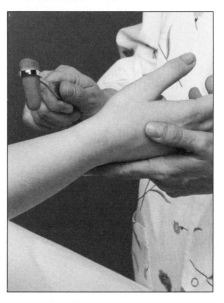

To test the patient's patellar reflex, position one hand under her knee, raising it slightly off the examination table. With your other hand, grasp the reflex hammer and strike the patient's patellar tendon just below the kneecap.

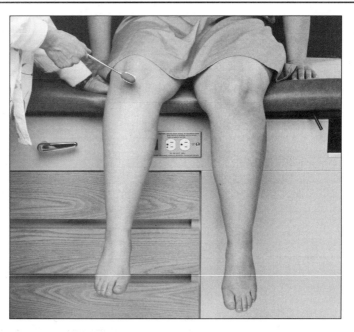

The leg should respond to your action by jerking forward.

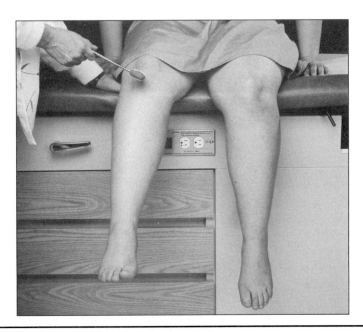

Next, test the Achilles tendon reflex. Hold the patient's foot in one hand and gently rotate the foot outward. Strike the Achilles tendon with the reflex hammer.

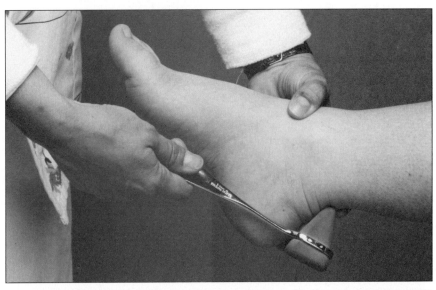

Watch for plantar flexion of the foot. The muscle should relax in 1 to 2 seconds.

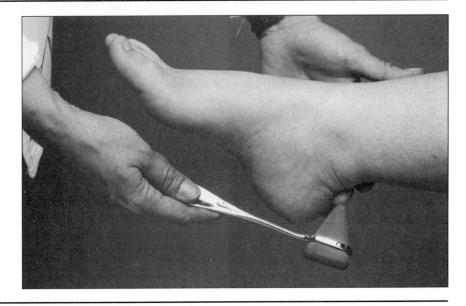

You can augment the reflexes by having the patient isometrically tense muscles not directly involved in the reflex arc being tested. For example, you might ask the patient to lock her fingers together and pull one hand against the other (Jendrassik's maneuver) while you try to elicit the patellar reflex by striking the knee with the hammer (as shown). This activity should elicit reflexes in the lower extremities.

To augment the reflex arcs in the upper extremities, you might ask the patient to clench her jaws or tense the quadriceps.

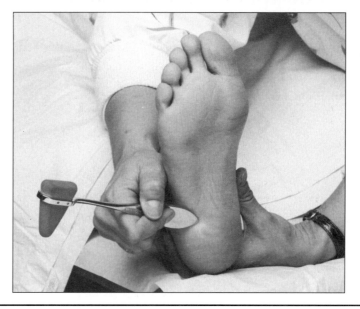

Testing the plantar reflex

To test this superficial reflex, use the handle of a reflex hammer to slowly stroke the lateral side of the patient's sole from the heel to the great toe.

The normal response is plantar flexion of the toes. Remember that this response may be diminished in older patients because of arthritic deformities of the foot or toes.

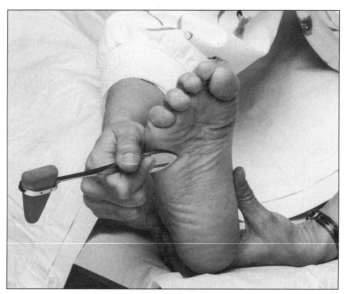

Testing primitive reflexes

If your patient has exhibited bilateral hyperactive reflexes or an abnormal plantar reflex, check her primitive reflexes: the grasp reflex and the snout reflex.

To elicit the grasp reflex, gently touch the patient's palm with your index and middle fingers.

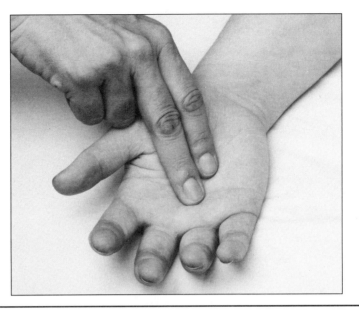

Flexion of the patient's fingers around yours, especially if she is otherwise unresponsive, is a positive grasp reflex.

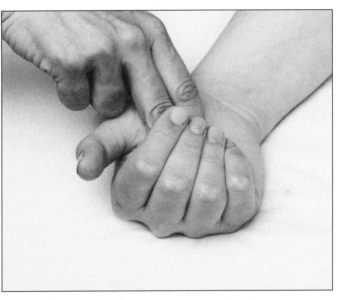

To test the snout reflex, sweep a tongue blade quickly and gently across the patient's lips. Move the tongue blade from side to side.

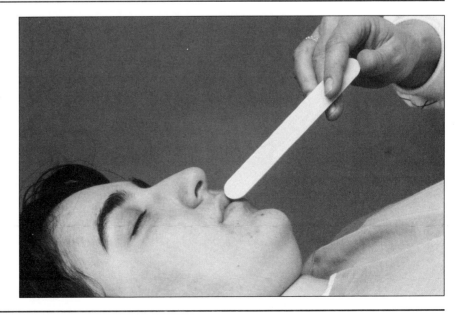

Observe for puckering of the lips, which is a positive snout reflex. Sucking movements of the lips and tongue indicate a positive sucking reflex. After you've completed your assessment, document your findings.

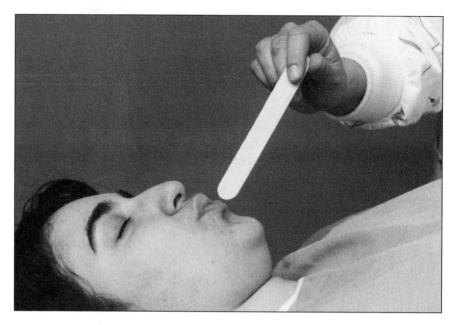

EXAMINING PERIPHERAL CIRCULATION

Because assessing your patient's peripheral vascular system provides information about blood circulation through the arteries, veins, and capillaries, you'll need to be familiar with the major vessels and pulse points before you begin your assessment. (See *Vascular structures.*)

Vascular structures

Below are the major arteries (red), veins (gray), and pulse points of the vascular system.

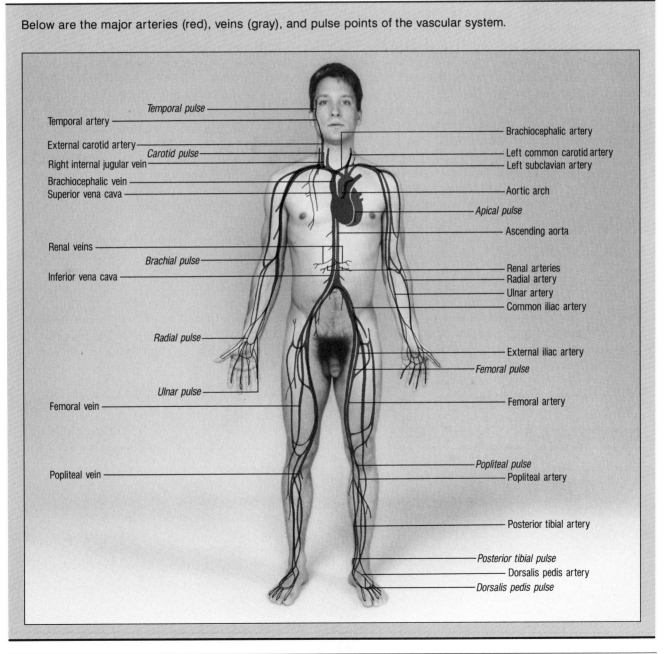

Temporal pulse
Temporal artery
External carotid artery
Carotid pulse
Right internal jugular vein
Brachiocephalic vein
Superior vena cava
Renal veins
Brachial pulse
Inferior vena cava
Radial pulse
Ulnar pulse
Femoral vein
Popliteal vein

Brachiocephalic artery
Left common carotid artery
Left subclavian artery
Aortic arch
Apical pulse
Ascending aorta
Renal arteries
Radial artery
Ulnar artery
Common iliac artery
External iliac artery
Femoral pulse
Femoral artery
Popliteal pulse
Popliteal artery
Posterior tibial artery
Posterior tibial pulse
Dorsalis pedis artery
Dorsalis pedis pulse

Lynne Patzek Miller, RN,C, BS, operating room manager at Doylestown (Pa.) Hospital, and *Teresa A. Palmer, RN, MSN, CANP*, a nurse practitioner in adult cardiac surgery at Robert Wood Johnson University Hospital, New Brunswick, N.J., contributed to this section. The publisher thanks *Hill-Rom*, Batesville, Ind., and *North Penn Hospital*, Lansdale, Pa., for their help.

REVIEWING THE VASCULAR SYSTEM

A vast network of blood vessels, the vascular system keeps blood circulating to and from every functioning cell in the body. This core network consists of arteries and veins and such extensions as capillaries.

The arteries carry oxygenated blood from the lungs to the heart and then to the body. The only artery that doesn't carry oxygenated blood is the pulmonary artery.

The main artery—the aorta—branches into vessels that supply specific organs or areas of the body. Three major branches arise from the arch of the aorta: the left common carotid, left subclavian, and left brachiocephalic arteries. These vessels take oxygen to the brain, arms, and upper chest. The descending aorta takes oxygen to GI and genitourinary organs, the spinal column, and the lower chest and abdominal muscles. From the abdominal area, the aorta forks into the iliac arteries, which further branch into the femoral arteries.

To complete the cycle, the venous system returns blood to the heart and then to the lungs for gas exchange and reoxygenation. The only vein that carries oxygenated blood is the pulmonary vein.

ASSESSING CIRCULATION

Your assessment of peripheral circulation typically begins as you take the patient's pulse. You can feel or hear the pressure wave of blood exiting the heart and surging through the arteries. Normally, you can palpate this recurring fluid wave—or pulse—at locations on the body where an artery crosses over bone or firm tissue. By assessing peripheral pulses, you can indirectly determine the status of peripheral arterial circulation.

To evaluate the peripheral vasculature, you'll perform inspection, palpation, and auscultation—with palpation as the primary tool for assessing blood flow to the extremities. To palpate pulses safely, apply gentle pressure to each pulse with the index and middle fingers of your dominant hand. Document the rate (beats/minute), rhythm (regular or irregular), amplitude (strength of contractions), and bilateral symmetry of each pulse.

One of the most telling signs of peripheral vascular health or disease is pulse amplitude—especially in such areas as the neck, arms, and legs. This sign reflects the vigor of left ventricular contractions and the patency of peripheral vessels. To evaluate pulse amplitude, use a numerical scale, a descriptive term, or another system favored by your hospital. The following numerical scale and the corresponding descriptions of pulse amplitude are in common use:

+3 — bounding (readily palpable, forceful, not easily obliterated by finger pressure)
+2 — normal (easily palpable and obliterated only by strong finger pressure)
+1 — weak or thready (hard to palpate and easily obliterated by slight finger pressure)
0 — absent (undiscernible).

Remember, only +2 describes a normal pulse.

To complement your physical assessment findings, you'll need to take a thorough health history. Ask the patient about factors that can significantly affect peripheral circulation. For example, ask about his job requirements, activities of daily living, and cardiovascular health and whether he has a history of diabetes. (See *Exploring circulatory complaints.*)

ASSESSMENT CHECKLIST

Exploring circulatory complaints

To detect potential abnormalities in peripheral circulation, conduct a thorough health history. If you think the patient's peripheral circulation may be impaired or if he voices related complaints, ask questions to elicit further information, as follows:

☐ Do you have a history of heart disease? If so, can you describe the problem?

☐ Do you have high blood pressure?

☐ Have you ever been diagnosed with an aortic aneurysm?

☐ Do you have a history of diabetes? If so, how long have you had it? Can you describe your treatment plan?

☐ Do your shoes or rings ever feel tight? Do your ankles or feet ever swell? If so, when does this occur?

☐ Have you noticed any change in feeling in your legs? If so, would you describe this feeling as numbness or pain? How long does this feeling last?

☐ Have you noticed any change in color in your legs or feet? If so, can you describe the change? When does it occur and how long does it last?

☐ Do you have any sores or ulcers on your legs or feet? If so, are they healing?

☐ What kinds of activities does your job require? Do your job duties include much standing or sitting in one place?

Preparing to assess peripheral circulation

Begin by assembling your equipment: gloves and a stethoscope.

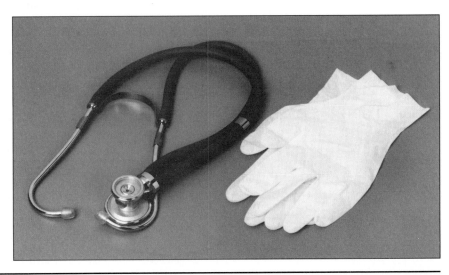

Wash your hands. Explain the procedure to the patient, answer any questions he may have, and provide reassurance. Then place him in a comfortable, relaxed position. Use the supine position if he can tolerate it: This position gives you easy access to all peripheral pulses.

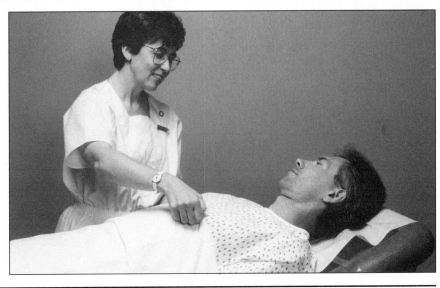

Inspecting the arms and legs

Observe the patient's arms and legs. Note the color of his skin (pink, pale, or cyanotic), and check closely for edema. If you observe edema, identify its location and check for symmetry. Note the location and size of any lesions, rashes, or scaly areas. Also assess hair patterns on the arms, legs, hands, and feet. (The presence of hair indicates an adequate arterial blood supply.)

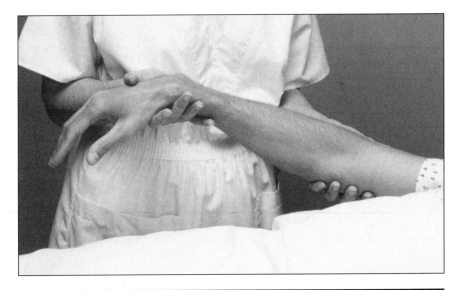

Observe the nail beds for normal growth. Note any thickening of the nails, an indicator of impaired circulation.

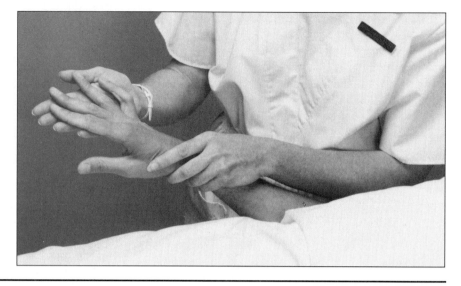

Palpating peripheral pulses

Palpate the skin on the arms and legs to determine its temperature (cold, cool, warm, or hot).

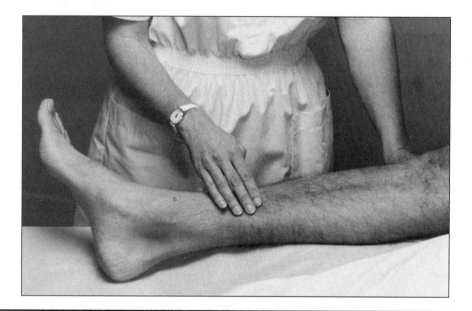

If you noticed any edema during inspection, determine its type (pitting or nonpitting) and degree (from +1 to +4). To do so, press the area firmly with your finger for 5 to 10 seconds, and then remove your finger. Note the extent and duration of a depression on the skin.

▶ *Clinical tip:* Pitting edema progresses in severity from +1 (a barely perceptible depression) to +4 (a persistent pit as deep as 1″ [2.5 cm]). The higher the score, the more significant the edema.

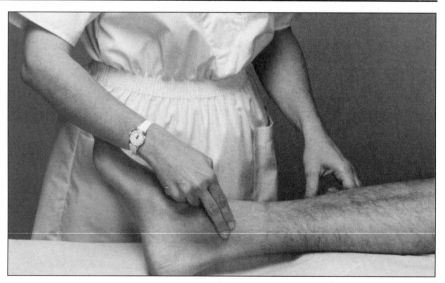

Squeeze the nail beds on all extremities to produce blanching. Note how much time passes before the nail bed color returns.

▶ *Clinical tip:* Normal capillary refill time is 3 seconds or less.

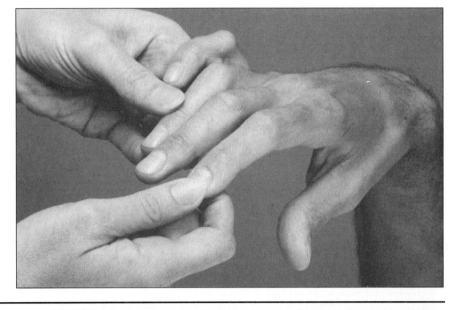

Next, palpate the peripheral pulses, beginning with the carotid pulse. Place your fingers lightly on the patient's neck just medial to the trachea and below the jaw angle (as shown). Repeat the action on the opposite side.

▶ *Clinical tip:* Palpate only one carotid artery at a time; simultaneous palpation can slow the pulse or decrease the blood pressure, causing the patient to faint.

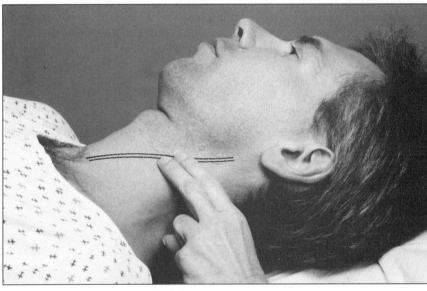

To palpate the brachial pulse, position your fingers in the groove between the biceps and the triceps muscle, just above the elbow. Repeat the action on the opposite arm.

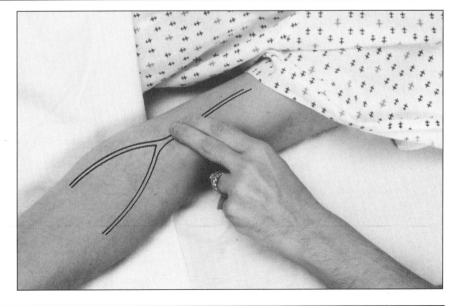

To palpate the radial pulse, place your fingers on the medial and ventral side of the wrist, in line with the thumb (as shown). Repeat the action on the opposite wrist.

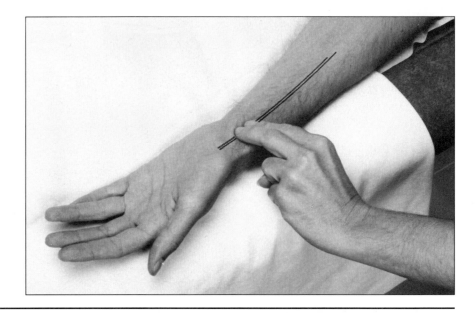

To palpate the femoral pulse, put on gloves, and press deeply about midway between the anterior superior iliac spine and the symphysis pubis (as shown). Repeat the action on the opposite side. (Then remove the gloves if you wish.)

▶ *Clinical tip:* In obese patients, palpate the crease of the groin, halfway between the pubic bone and the hip bone.

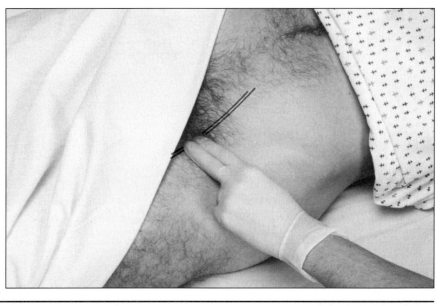

To palpate the popliteal pulse, flex the patient's knee. Press the fingers of both hands deeply into the popliteal fossa at the back of the knee. Repeat the action on the opposite knee.

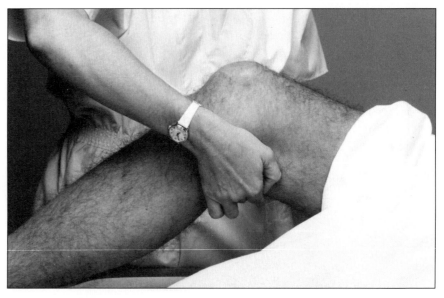

If you can't palpate the popliteal pulse with the patient in the position described above, reposition him onto his abdomen (if he can tolerate this position). Press deeply into the popliteal fossa to palpate the pulse (as shown).

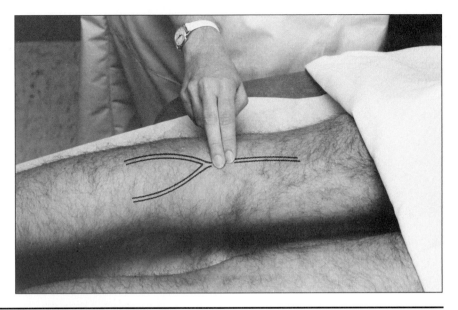

To palpate the posterior tibial pulse, apply pressure slightly below the medial malleolus of the ankle. Repeat the action on the opposite ankle.

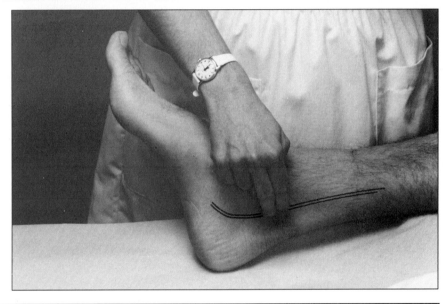

To palpate the dorsalis pedis pulse, position your fingers in the medial dorsum of the foot, just lateral to the extensor tendon of the great toe. If the pulse is difficult to palpate, instruct the patient to point his toes downward. Repeat the action on the opposite foot.

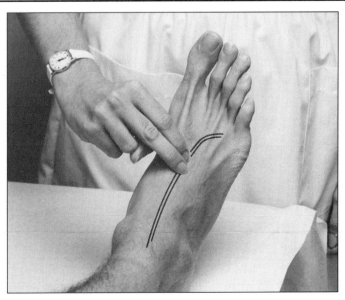

Auscultating peripheral pulses with a stethoscope

If you can locate peripheral pulses with palpation alone, proceed to auscultate blood flow with a stethoscope. Place the bell of the stethoscope over the carotid artery (as shown), and ask the patient to hold his breath. Listen for vascular sounds (such as murmurs or bruits). Repeat the action on the opposite side. Normally, you should hear no vascular sounds over the peripheral arteries. Vascular sounds in these areas may indicate a central circulation problem.

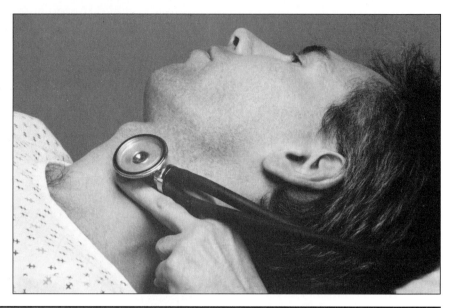

After putting on gloves, locate the femoral artery and place the bell of the stethoscope over the site. Listen for vascular sounds; then repeat the action on the opposite side. (Afterward, you may remove the gloves if you wish.)

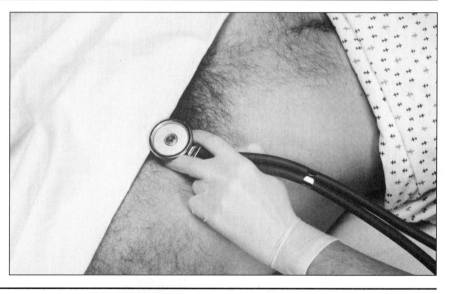

Place the bell of the stethoscope over the popliteal pulse site. Listen for vascular sounds. Repeat the action on the opposite side.

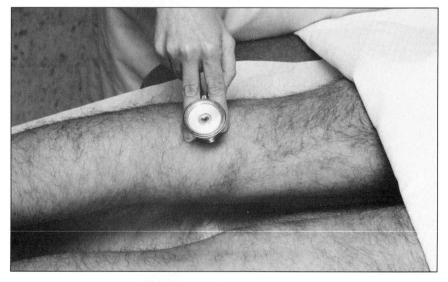

Auscultating peripheral pulses with ultrasound

If you can't locate peripheral pulses by palpation alone, use a Doppler ultrasound stethoscope to locate pulses and auscultate blood flow. Apply a small amount of coupling gel (not water-soluble lubricant) to the area being assessed and on the head of the ultrasound transducer (a sensitive wandlike component that amplifies the sound of blood flowing through the vessels and that can convert ultrasonic waves to electrical impulses).

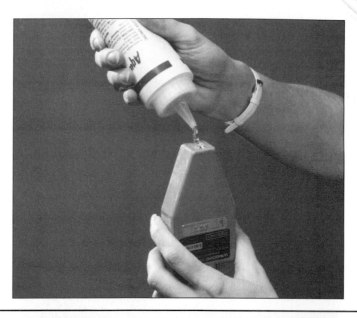

Turn the volume-control knob counterclockwise to the lowest audible setting while depressing the ON button (as shown). Adjust the volume so that you receive a clear amplification of the pulse.

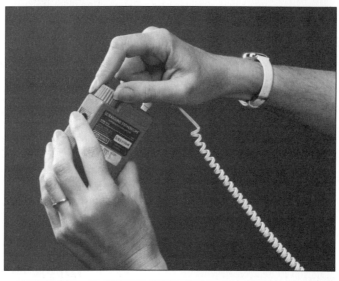

Position the transducer on the skin directly over the selected artery. Then angle the transducer about 45 degrees from the artery, making sure that the gel comes between the skin and the transducer. Move the transducer slowly in a circular motion until you locate the center of the artery. This positioning will help you obtain a clear, pulsating sound.

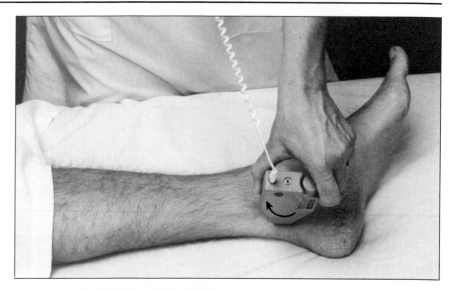

Count the sign pulse rate. Wipe
to determine 60 seconds
away any from the pulse site
with a gauze pad, and mark the
spots where you heard the pulse.
This will help you relocate the
pulse if necessary.

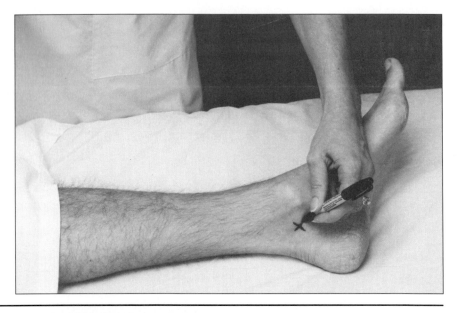

Then clean the head of the transducer with a clean gauze pad.
Document all findings on the patient's assessment flow sheet. Report any abnormal findings to the
doctor.

▶ *Clinical tip:* When cleaning
the head of the transducer,
don't use alcohol or an abrasive
cleaner. These substances can
damage the head, interfering with
sound transmission.

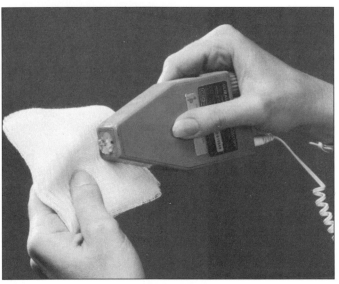

INDEX